# Evaluating the Impact of Implementing Evidence-Based Practice

Edited by

Debra Bick and
Ian D. Graham

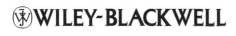

WILEY-BLACKWELL

A John Wiley & Sons, Ltd., Publication

Sigma Theta Tau International
Honor Society of Nursing®

This edition first published 2010
© 2010 by Sigma Theta Tau International

Blackwell Publishing was acquired by John Wiley & Sons in February 2007. Blackwell's publishing programme has been merged with Wiley's global Scientific, Technical, and Medical business to form Wiley-Blackwell.

*Registered office*
John Wiley & Sons Ltd, The Atrium, Southern Gate, Chichester, West Sussex, PO19 8SQ, United Kingdom

*Editorial offices*
9600 Garsington Road, Oxford, OX4 2DQ, United Kingdom
2121 State Avenue, Ames, Iowa 50014-8300, USA

For details of our global editorial offices, for customer services and for information about how to apply for permission to reuse the copyright material in this book please see our website at www.wiley.com/wiley-blackwell.

The right of the author to be identified as the author of this work has been asserted in accordance with the UK Copyright, Designs and Patents Act 1988.

*Library of Congress Cataloging-in-Publication Data*
Evaluating the impact of implementing evidence-based practice / edited by Debra Bick and Ian D. Graham.
 p. ; cm. – (Evidence based nursing series)
 Includes bibliographical references and index.
 ISBN 978-1-4051-8384-0 (pbk. : alk. paper)
 1. Evidence-based nursing. I. Bick. Debra. II. Graham, Ian D. III. Sigma Theta Tau International. IV. Series. Evidence-based nursing series.
 [DNLM: 1. Evidence-Based Nursing. 2. Evidence-Based Medicine. 3. Program Evaluation–methods. 4. Treatment outcome. WY 100.7 E92 2010]
 RT84.5.E927 2010
 610.73—dc22
 2009046229

A catalogue record for this book is available from the British Library.

Set in 11/13pt Sabon by MPS Limited, A Macmillan Company
Printed and bound in Malaysia by Vivar Printing Sdn Bhd

1   2010

The *Evidence-Based Nursing Series*

The *Evidence-Based Nursing Series* is co-published with Sigma Theta Tau International (STTI). The series focuses on implementing evidence-based practice in nursing and midwifery, and mirrors the remit of *Worldviews on Evidence-Based Nursing*, encompassing clinical practice, administration, research and public policy.

Other titles in the *Evidence-Based Nursing Series*:

**Models and Frameworks for Implementing Evidence-Based Practice: Linking Evidence to Action**
Edited by Jo Rycroft-Malone and Tracey Bucknall
ISBN: 978-1-4051-7594-4

**Clinical Context for Evidence-Based Nursing Practice**
Edited by Bridie Kent and Brendan McCormack
ISBN: 978-1-4051-8433-5

# Contents

# Contributors' information

*Debra Bick*

Debra Bick (RM, BA, MedSci, PhD) was appointed Professor of Evidence Based Midwifery Practice at King's College London in September 2008. Debra's research interests include maternal physical and psychological morbidity, the content and organization of services for postnatal women and their families, approaches to evidence synthesis and transfer and factors affecting clinical decision making. She is Editor-in-Chief of "Midwifery: An International Journal," Visiting Professor at the University of Sao Paulo, and Visiting Fellow at Bournemouth University. Her current research projects include the Hospital to Home postnatal care study and PEARLS a UK-wide matched pair cluster trial of a training intervention to enhance perineal trauma outcomes. She is a collaborator on an NIHR RfPB funded trial of diamorphine compared with pethidine for pain relief during labor and an NIHR HTA funded trial of upright compared with supine positions in the second stage of labor in primiparous women who have epidural analgesia. She was also a collaborator on two recently completed NIHR SDO projects on protocol-based care which highlighted a number of important issues for EBP.

*Barbara Davies*

Barbara Davies (RN PhD) is Associate Professor, School of Nursing, University of Ottawa, Canada, and is the Co-Director of the Nursing Best Practice Research Unit, a partnership with the Registered Nurses' Association of Ontario. She is the Site Director at Ottawa of the Ontario Training Centre for Health Services and Policy Research and co-teaches an interprofessional distance graduate course entitled Knowledge Transfer. She holds a Premier's Research Excellence Award for a program of research entitled *Interventions to promote successful sustained research transfer in nursing practice and health care.*

## Diane M. Doran

Diane Doran (RN, PhD, FCAHS) is a full Professor at the Lawrence S. Bloomberg Faculty of Nursing, University of Toronto where she also holds a Ministry of Health and Long-Term Care Nursing Senior Researcher Award. She is an adjunct professor at the School of Nursing, Queens University, and the School of Nursing, University of Technology, Sydney, Australia. She is Director of the Nursing Health Services Research Unit, University of Toronto. Dr Doran has recognized expertise in outcomes measurement, patient safety, knowledge translation, and e-Health.

## Nancy Edwards

Nancy Edwards is a Professor, School of Nursing and Department of Epidemiology and Community Medicine, University of Ottawa. She is an Associate Scientist, Elisabeth-Bruyere Research Institute, a Principal Scientist, Institute of Population Health and a Fellow of the Canadian Academy of Health Sciences. Dr. Edwards is also Scientific Director, Canadian Institutes of Health Research, Institute of Population and Public Health. She holds a Nursing Chair funded by the Canadian Health Services Research Foundation, the Canadian Institutes of Health Research and the Government of Ontario. Her research interests are in the area of multi-strategy and multi-level interventions in community health. She is leading programs of research in Canada and internationally.

## Christina Godfrey

Christina Godfrey (BA (Hons) (Psychology), BNSc (Nursing), MSc (Nursing)) is currently enrolled as a PhD candidate in the School of Rehabilitation Science, Queen's University. Specializing in the methodo-logy of synthesis and integrative research, Christina has received comprehensive training (Cochrane & Joanna Briggs Institute), and is co-author of both quantitative and qualitative systematic reviews. Christina continues in her role of Assistant Director of the Queen's Joanna Briggs Collaboration and is currently teaching methodology at the graduate level in her role as adjunct faculty, Queen's University School of Nursing.

## Lisa Gold

Lisa Gold (MA Cantab (Economics), MSc Oxon (Economics for Development)) is a Senior Research Fellow at Deakin Health Economics, Deakin University, Australia. Lisa is a health economist with over 10 years experience in the economic evaluation of maternal and child public health and social interventions to improve population health and reduce health inequalities. She has also conducted systematic reviews of evidence and methodological development in economic evaluation in the UK and Australia. Her research interests focus on the evaluation of complex and community-based interventions and the use of stated preference methods to explore individual and community values for such interventions.

### Ian D. Graham

Ian Graham obtained a PhD in medical sociology from McGill University. He took leave from his position as an Associate Professor in the School of Nursing at the University of Ottawa to assume the position of Vice President of Knowledge Translation at the Canadian Institutes of Health Research. His research has largely focused on knowledge translation (the process of research use) and conducting applied research on strategies to increase implementation of research findings and EBP. He has studied adaptation, implementation, and quality appraisal of practice guidelines, as well as the uptake of guidelines and decision support tools by practitioners. He has also studied researchers' and health research funding agencies' KT activities, the determinants of research use, and theories/models of planned change.

### Margaret B. Harrison

Margaret B. Harrison (RN PhD) is a Professor at the School of Nursing, and cross-appointed with the Department of Community Health and Epidemiology at Queen's University. She is a Senior Scientist with the Practice and Research in Nursing Group (PRN) at Queen's University, an innovative academic-practice partnership to advance research at the point of care. She is also Director of the Queen's Joanna Briggs Collaboration, the first North American partner of the Joanna Briggs Institute, a sister organization to Cochrane, engaged in advancing syntheses of all types of evidence. Dr Harrison is a founding member of the international ADAPTE collaboration, a group that is focused on development and testing a rigorous methodology to develop guidelines for different contexts.

Her research program is focused continuity of care for complex health populations and EBP—themes which are intertwined. Knowledge translation and implementation of guidelines is an important strategy for improving continuity. She has worked with pan-Canadian organizations such as the Stroke Network and the Cancer Partnership, as well as more local and regional bodies reorganizing care based on evidence. Her research crosses community, hospital, and long-term care sectors, and she has received support from provincial (MOHLTC, OHSF) and national funding councils (NHRDP, CIHR, SSHRC).

## Neil Johnson

Neil Johnson (RGN, BA (Hons), PGCTLT, MSc) is a Lecturer in adult nursing at the Robert Gordon University, School of Nursing and Midwifery, Aberdeen. At present Neil teaches within both undergraduate and postgraduate programs and has been involved in a variety of projects exploring the implementation of evidence in practice and impacts from evidence in practice. At present Neil is evaluating the use of practice manuals in nursing.

## Anne Sales

Anne Sales (RN PhD) is a Professor in the Faculty of Nursing, University of Alberta, Canada Research Chair in Interdisciplinary Healthcare Teams, and Chair in Primary Care Research. She has conducted 19 funded research projects, focusing on improving quality of care, knowledge translation, and implementation of evidence-based best practice, and has over 65 peer-reviewed publications. Her training is in sociology, health economics, econometrics, and general health services research. She is currently conducting two studies of audit with feedback interventions, one in long-term care settings, the other in acute hospital and primary care settings.

## Sharon E. Straus

Sharon Straus (MD, MSc, FRCPC) is a geriatrician/general internist/ clinical epidemiologist. She is an Associate Professor in the Department of Medicine at the University of Toronto. She is the Director of the Knowledge Translation Program, Li Ka Shing Knowledge Institute at St Michael's Hospital and the University of Toronto. Her research interests include mentorship and the evaluation of interventions to facilitate knowledge translation and promote quality of care.

She holds more than $18 million in peer-reviewed grants from the CIHR, CHSRF, and the Premier's Research Excellence Award amongst others. She was awarded a Canada Research Chair in Knowledge Translation and a Health Scholar Award from the Alberta Heritage Foundation for Medical Research.

## Jacqueline Tetroe

Jacqueline Tetroe has a Masters Degree in developmental psychology and studied cognitive and educational psychology at the

Ontario Institute for Studies in Education. She currently works as a senior advisor in Knowledge Translation at the Canadian Institutes of Health Research. Her research interests focus on the process of knowledge translation and on strategies to increase the uptake and implementation of EBP as well as to increase the understanding of the barriers and facilitators that impact on successful implementation. She is a strong advocate of the use of conceptual models to both guide and interpret research.

### Dominique Tremblay

Dominique Tremblay is a Canadian Health Services Research Foundation Postdoctoral Fellow. Her professional background is in clinical, first-line, and senior management of nursing services. She completed a PhD in nursing administration at University of Montreal and currently conducting her postdoctoral research program with Dr Nancy Edwards at the University of Ottawa. Her research interests focus on the translation process of innovative multiple interventions in cancer services using mixed methods research design. EBP and outcomes of EBP relate to her domain of interest representing a typical case of an innovative intervention involving multiple actors, multiple strategies, and multiple levels of the health care system.

### Joyce E. Wilkinson

Joyce E. Wilkinson (PhD, BA, DipCPCouns, RSCN, RGN) is RHV Research Fellow, Social Dimensions of Health Institute, University of St Andrews. Her research interests include RU/KU/EBP implementation processes and evaluation of impacts and outcomes of RU/KU/EBPI.

### Peter Wimpenny

Peter Wimpenny (RGN, BSc (Hons), Cert Ed, PhD) is the Associate Director of the Joanna Briggs Collaborating Centre in Aberdeen, Scotland, based at the Robert Gordon University. He has had involvement and interest in EBP for some years. He was a member of SIGN (Scottish Intercollegiate Guideline Network) Council from 2001 to 2006 and actively involved in a number of projects exploring guideline development and implementation. At present he is involved in a variety of EBP-related work that includes systematic reviews, evaluation of use of practice manuals, and development of summarized evidence for community staff as part of the Joanna Briggs Institute.

# Foreword

The arrival of the evidence-based 'movement' emerged at a particular moment in history when faith in technocratic and scientific rationalism in policy circles seemed to reach its apotheosis. What this book demonstrates so compellingly is that this 'movement' was the product of the convergence of ideas, individuals, institutions and infrastructure as well as policy drivers. It is hard to imagine the global spread of this endeavour and its embedding within health-care without the use of the internet but, in evaluating the impact of implementing evidence-based practice, this book reveals what a sophisticated science evidence-based practice has become. Most of all, it shows the importance of under-pinning implementation of evidence with a change management strategy. The story of EBP is well told – its impetus lies in the desire to improve outcomes for patients by implementing those that were clinically effective and cost-effective, eliminating those practices that did not meet the criteria. The apostle of this new movement was Archie Cochrane, whose name christened the collaboration that now represents arguably the most authoritative and largest methodological evidence synthesis industry globally. Cochrane also advocated the application of EBP to education, social work, criminology and social policy, which is now being taken forward by the Campbell Collaboration. However, under the leadership of Sir Iain Chalmers and colleagues at the National Perinatal Epidemiology Unit in Oxford, it was pregnancy and childbirth that blazed the trail, starting in the late 1970s through the development of stringent standards for the evaluation of evidence and the development of EBP. Fuelled partly by impatience with the vagaries of evidence, its implementation, as well as a sense of moral outrage at persistent inequalities in outcomes, Chalmers and colleagues created an encyclopaedia of evidence that became the landmark reference in the field. In the early 1990s, Chalmers turned his attention to establishing the international Cochrane Collaboration. A prominent part of the early EBP movement was support from consumers and the user voice continues to be given due prominence by the Collaboration.

The epicentre of the EBP movement in the UK was Oxford in the mid-1980s, where acolytes such as David Sackett congregated and spread the word from cognate initiatives across the Atlantic; Canada in particular. The influence of EBP quickly spread to the UK and Australia. It was not just that the use of evidence and measures of rigour and quality promulgated, which was itself new, but a new urgency coalesced that the clinical- and cost-effectiveness of health-care interventions needed to be considered. Concurrent initiatives within the UK National Health Service, including the development of the NHS Library and Information service founded by Sir Muir Gray provided infrastructure, and the establishment of the National Institute for Health and Clinical Excellence and the Centre for Reviews and Dissemination, University of York in the UK, were tasked to sieve the evidence and turn it into guidelines. David Sackett, and Jonathan Lomas from Canada became synonymous with the success of the movement, which swiftly spawned further branches of activity, including research utilization, knowledge transfer and exchange, knowledge translation and implementation science. Similarly, as this book reveals, the embedding of the approach within nursing, specifically cardiovascular nursing and allied health professions, has impacted albeit in a patchy manner. The value and utility of the effort invested in EBP lies not only in putting the evidence into the hands of clinicians, turning that into better outcomes for patients in a cost-effective manner, but also in developing the mechanisms and conditions to do so. This volume not only pulls the evidence together from key leaders and experts in the field of implementation nationally, but also internationally. The resulting synthesis summarizes the state of the science but also reveals that outcomes rely upon multi-layered and multi-faceted interventions, and a skill set that stretches from the academic to advocacy and political mobilization. Politics is never far from the surface in this gripping tale. We might explain the rise of EBP as the desire on the part of policy makers to distance themselves from the dilemmas of allocating resources in health-care and the evidence presented here reveals the unintended consequences and challenges of sustaining impacts along the way. This book has the rare virtue of not taking us round the reflexive loop of only providing the tools to evaluate outcomes of implementation. It advises on what needs to be considered when making change and on what will make that change stick.

Professor Anne Marie Rafferty
*BSc MPhil DPhil (Oxon) RGN DN FRCN*
*Head of School*
*Florence Nightingale School of Nursing & Midwifery*
*King's College London*

# Preface

As a consequence of evidence-based practice (EBP), many of us reside in countries where there have been tremendous changes in approaches to clinical education and skills training, patient care, and funding of our health services. EBP evolved from recognition that many areas of clinical care were unsupported by evidence of clinical or cost-effectiveness, with continued use of unproven interventions relying in many cases on an assumption of benefit. Once an area of practice had been questioned and evidence of impact became available, it was clear that interventions which did not result in benefit or could lead to harm should be withdrawn. Conversely, interventions associated with improved outcomes should be universally implemented. The role of EBP in informing the provision and content of 21st century health care is now a policy priority, a move which has triggered ongoing public debate about the role of politics in health care.

As researchers, contributors to national policy guidance, members of funding bodies, and educators, we have followed recent debates with interest. What stimulated us to produce this book was recognition of the continuing gap between use of evidence and impact on outcomes. Despite the drive to implement EBP, there is still limited guidance on how to assess if implementation was effective, the issues which should be considered or range of approaches which could be used to measure outcomes. Work to date which has addressed implementation has often measured success in terms of whether a specific clinical outcome was or was not achieved, and has not considered other impacts, some of which may not have occurred immediately (such as whether an intervention was sustained in practice) or may have occurred at other points along the pathway of implementation (such as clinician or patient behavior change). Detrimental practices persist despite a plethora of systematic reviews and tools to assist implementation such as guidelines and protocols. This may be due to poor implementation of the evidence in the first instance, failure to sustain successful implementation, lack of robust evaluation of implementation processes and outcomes, or failure to consider the range of impacts (intended and unintended) which may have occurred.

Our contributors have all had "hands-on" experience of contributing to or leading on studies of implementation of EBP and bring together a wealth of research experience. We appreciate that work related to evaluation of outcomes is developing and that funding bodies and policy makers are crucial to taking this work forward. In the interim, we hope that this book will stimulate those involved with the development, implementation, and evaluation of EBP to appreciate that equal priority needs to be accorded to how outcomes of implementation are derived, measured, and reported on.

Debra Bick and
Ian D. Graham

# Chapter 1

# The importance of addressing outcomes of evidence-based practice

*Debra Bick and Ian D. Graham*

---

**Key learning points**

- Most of us reside in countries where healthcare resources are finite but healthcare costs and demands are increasing.
- Health service funders, providers, and policy makers need to ensure interventions associated with evidence of shorter- and longer-term clinical and cost-effectiveness are implemented. This is often hindered by a lack of information on what comprises a "good" or a "bad" outcome from the perspectives of relevant stakeholders.
- Use of evidence-based practice (EBP) is assumed to lead to better health outcomes; however, it is clear that use of tools such as guidelines, protocols, and pathways may not lead to anticipated benefits if all relevant outcomes, including process outcomes, are not considered from the outset.
- Despite the development of models and theoretical frameworks to support EBP, implementation remains a complex undertaking. Interventions to support the use of EBP need to reflect context, culture, and facilitation.
- Approaches to derive and evaluate outcomes need to be undertaken with the same level of rigor as other interventions and procedures that the EBP movement focuses on.

## Introduction

In this chapter, the background to the development of the book is outlined as are some of the reasons why we felt it was timely and appropriate to bring together a text which focuses on the outcomes of implementation of evidence-based practice (EBP). Experts in the field of knowledge translation and EBP invited to contribute chapters to the book were asked to consider how to determine if outcomes of EBP in their areas of expertise were efficacious, how efficacy could be measured, and how to ascertain if the outcomes of interest were the most important from the perspectives of relevant stakeholders. As described by Ian Graham and colleagues in Chapter 2, outcomes of EBP could include change in behavior demonstrating use of evidence in practice and impact of use on outcomes such as better health and more effective use of healthcare resources.

## Why are outcomes of EBP important?

We hope that by reading the chapters and following the perspectives presented by the authors that the need to accord equal priority to the outcomes of implementation as with all other steps to support the use of research in practice will become apparent. Most of us live in countries where healthcare resources are finite, an issue whether our healthcare is largely funded through our taxes or private insurance schemes. Some readers will reside in countries where healthcare systems face an unprecedented increase in the burden of ill health arising from chronic, non-communicable diseases—for example as a consequence of the epidemic of obesity or an aging population. Others will reside in countries which face epidemics of disease including TB, HIV/AIDS, persistent high maternal and infant mortality and morbidity, or where poor or fractured infrastructure cannot support an effective healthcare system. For those living in developed countries, while there have been unprecedented advances in healthcare technology and year on year increases in healthcare funding from government, the increase in resources has not been matched by improvements in health. This is most evident in the US, where it is estimated that healthcare costs for 2009 were $2.7 trillion, the highest level of healthcare spend anywhere in the world, yet life expectancy is lower than in many other developed and middle-income countries indicating large discrepancies between healthcare costs and outcomes (Institute of Medicine 2009). We also have healthcare systems where despite a plethora of technology, gaps remain in the quality of data to accurately inform and compare the outcomes of care. In the UK, efforts to gauge whether investment in healthcare following the election of a Labour government in 1997 had resulted in improved health outcomes were hampered by constraints in measures of quality and need for better measures of output and outcome extending beyond hospital episode data (Lakhani et al. 2005).

## The development of EBP

For the last two decades, in response to some of the reasons outlined above, greater emphasis has been placed on the need to provide healthcare informed by evidence of effectiveness, the premise being that use of evidence will optimize health outcomes for the service user and maximize use of finite healthcare resources. The main drivers for EBP have come from political and policy initiatives which also instigated the establishment of organizations to develop guidance to inform healthcare such as the National Institute for Health and Clinical Effectiveness (NICE) in England and Wales, the Scottish Intercollegiate Guideline Network, and the US Agency for Healthcare Research and Quality. The remit of a national body such as NICE is to make recommendations for care based on best evidence of clinical and cost-effectiveness. Suites of guidelines to inform a range of acute and chronic physical and psychological health conditions and appraisals of innovations in technology and pharmacology have been developed and published by NICE which aim to standardize patient care, reduce variation in health outcomes, discourage use of interventions with no proven efficacy, and encourage systematic assessment of patient outcomes. The National Institute for Health Research which funds research to inform National Health Service (NHS) care in England requires studies funded across all of its programs to provide evidence of clinical and cost-effectiveness.

The role of NICE in the synthesis and dissemination of evidence to prioritize healthcare interventions has generated criticism that it promotes rationing in healthcare (Maynard et al. 2004), an issue with implications for determining how outcome measures are derived to elicit benefit and from whose perspective. As Maynard and colleagues (2004) write "...rationing is the inevitable corollary of prioritization, and NICE must fully inform rationing in the NHS," the issue being not *whether* but *how* to ration (p. 227). In the UK, publication of NICE guidance which does not support the use of a particular drug or therapy because the evidence reviewed did not indicate clinical or cost-effectiveness has frequently been challenged by industry (Maynard & Bloor 2009), service user charities, and in media reports of an individual's experience of being refused treatment which did not comply with NICE recommendations. Recent NICE recommendations which generated criticism about its role include restrictions on use of the drugs for people with early stage Alzheimer's disease, restrictions to fertility treatments, and use of drugs to treat kidney cancer. In some instances, the Department of Health was forced to reverse the original NICE recommendation to deflect public criticism, for example the use of Herceptin for women with early stage breast cancer (Lancet 2005). Nevertheless, this is an interesting juxtaposition—whose outcomes should receive the highest priority when decisions about healthcare interventions and optimal use of finite resources are made? That certain treatments may make a difference to someone's quality of life will not influence recommendation for use across the NHS if the evidence assessed does not demonstrate clinical or cost-effectiveness at thresholds set by NICE. The recent introduction of "top up" fees to enable patients to bypass NICE recommendations and purchase drugs not recommended for NHS use reflects the power of today's informed healthcare consumer (Gubb 2008). Although only likely to be utilized by a small group of people, as Maynard and Bloor (2009) propose, this raises issues about the role of NICE and regulation of the pharmaceutical industry; how drug prices should be determined; and how, if at all, to deal differently with rare or end-of-life conditions when making resource allocation decisions in healthcare. It also introduces the issue of consumers opting to purchase interventions which they view as likely to provide a better outcome which could include aspects of physical and/or psychological health and/or well-being.

The development of strategies to encourage use of evidence to inform decisions about healthcare was stimulated initially by what has been referred to as a "movement" for evidence-based medicine (EBM). One of the first people to propose that medical care should be informed by evidence of effectiveness was Archie Cochrane, whose book *Effectiveness and Efficiency: Random Reflections on Health Services* was published in 1972. Cochrane also advocated that this approach should be applied to education, social work, criminology, and social policy (Cochrane 1972). The work of Archie

Cochrane triggered groups such as those led by Gordon Guyatt and David Sackett to develop methods to synthesize and critique evidence to support decisions in clinical practice. In the late 1970s and 1980s, Ian Chalmers at the National Perinatal Epidemiology Unit in Oxford pioneered the methodology to systematically review the evidence related to effective care in pregnancy and childbirth. Building on this work, the Cochrane Centre was established in 1992 and was crucial for the spread of EBM, which in turn stimulated revisions to healthcare education and training, policy development, publication of new journals, and establishment of academic centers. Principles of EBM have subsequently been applied to support the commissioning of healthcare services, recommendations for pharmacology treatments, surgical interventions, diagnostic tests, and medical devices. Of note is that although attention has been paid to the use of measures of "outcome," limited attention has been paid to the definition or consequences of a "good" or "poor" outcome. Reviewers for the Cochrane Pregnancy and Childbirth group define an outcome as an "adverse health event" (Hofmeyr et al. 2008). In a Cochrane review, data from meta-analyses of relevant trials will be presented in a forest plot with the beneficial effect of an intervention presented to the left of the "no effect" line and a harmful effect to the right of the line. This is an extremely useful way to present outcomes of pooled data, but it is one part of the picture if we are to ensure that outcomes are the most relevant for all concerned. Further exploration of outcomes is required in order that consequences beyond implementation can be considered from a range of perspectives, an important stage in the continuum of research use.

## What is evidence?

There is ongoing debate as to the definition of "evidence" and what counts as evidence, although it seems consensus has been reached that evidence can come from a number of sources and not just the findings of randomized controlled trials (RCTs). A recent position paper from Sigma Theta Tau describes research evidence as:

> methodologically sound, clinically relevant research about the effectiveness and safety of interventions, the accuracy and precision of assessment measures, the power of prognostic markers, the

strength of causal relationships, the cost-effectiveness of nursing interventions, and the meaning of illness or patient experiences.

(Sigma Theta Tau International 2005–2007, Research and Scholarship Advisory Committee Position Statement 2008, p. 57)

In a 1996 commentary in the *British Medical Journal*, Sackett et al. (1996) defined EBM as "the conscientious, explicit, and judicious use of current best evidence in making decisions about the care of individual patients," and stressed the need for the clinician to use evidence along with their expertise and judgment to make decisions which also reflected the choice of the individual patient. A later *British Medical Journal* commentary reiterated that evidence alone should not be the main driver to change practice and that preferences and values needed to be explicit in clinical decision making (Guyatt et al. 2004). Of note is that the authors highlighted that the biggest future challenge for EBM was knowledge translation (Guyatt et al. 2004). The need to synthesize evidence for use by busy clinicians, to place evidence in a "hierarchy" with the most robust evidence at the top of the hierarchy and acknowledgment that evidence can come from a number of external sources continues to be emphasized (Bellomo and Bagshaw 2006).

When reading any literature which refers to use of evidence, it is apparent that a number of terms have been used to describe the process which include EBM, EBP, evidence-based clinical decision making and evidence-informed practice. The term *evidence-based practice* is more commonly used to describe evidence use by nurses, midwives, and members of the allied health professions (Sigma Theta Tau International Position Statement 2008).

Throughout this book, we refer to EBP in line with the following definition:

> the process of shared decision making between practitioner, patient, and others significant to them based on research evidence, the patient's experiences and preferences, clinical expertise or know-how, and other available robust sources of information.

(Rycroft-Malone et al. 2004)

As we have already indicated, an outcome could reflect behavior change at the individual, team, or organizational level, an improvement in individual health status or better use of healthcare resources.

The increase in access to electronic bibliographic databases, such as the Cochrane Library of Systematic Reviews, and dissemination strategies originally adopted by groups such as NICE, professional organizations, and healthcare providers were viewed as ways to increase clinician awareness of research, with an assumption that the use of research evidence would spontaneously occur and improved health patient outcomes would follow. Studies of dissemination and implementation strategies found that few were effective (Grimshaw et al. 2004). Grimshaw and colleagues (2004) undertook a systematic review of the effectiveness and efficiency of guideline dissemination and implementation strategies. Studies were selected for inclusion if they were RCTs, controlled clinical trials, controlled before and after studies, and interrupted time series. A total of 235 studies which looked at 309 comparisons met inclusion criteria. Overall study quality was poor. Multifaceted interventions were addressed in 73% of the comparisons. The majority of comparisons which reported dichotomous outcome data (87%) found some differences in outcomes with considerable variation in observed effects both within and across interventions. Single interventions which were commonly evaluated included reminders, dissemination of educational materials and audit and feedback. The majority of studies only reported costs of treatment, and only 25 studies reported costs of guideline development, dissemination or implementation although data presented in most cases was of low quality and not suitable for extraction for the review. In conclusion, the authors recommended that decision makers needed to use considerable judgment when making decisions about how best to use limited resources to maximum population health.

## Models and frameworks to support research use

A number of models and theoretical frameworks to support research use in practice have been developed—for example, the IOWA model (Titler et al. 2001), the PARiHS framework (Kitson et al. 1998) and the Ottawa Model (Graham & Logan 2004) which are described further in Chapter 3 of this book and are the focus of Book 1 of this series (Rycroft-Malone & Bucknall, 2010). It is now appreciated that implementation is complex, multifaceted, and multilayered and interventions need to be able to reflect and take account of context, culture, and facilitation to support and sustain research use.

Despite the development of frameworks and models as Helfrich and colleagues (2009) highlight with respect to PARiHS, there is as yet no pool of validated measures to operationalize the constructs defined in the framework. Work in this area is ongoing, as is other work to support research use including tools to assess the extent to which an organization is ready to adopt change. An example of this is the organization readiness to change assessment (ORCA) instrument developed by the Veterans Health Administration (VHA) Quality Enhancement Research Initiative for Ischemic Heart Disease (Helfrich et al. 2009). Although still in the developmental stage, this could be a useful approach for future implementation strategies.

## Why is it important to measure/evaluate the impact of EBP?

As illustrated in the following chapters that describe examples ranging from evaluation of outcomes of wound care interventions, cardiac care interventions, and the perspectives of service users, the importance of evaluating the outcomes of use of evidence is essential. The need to submit the evaluation of outcomes to the same level of rigor as other interventions and procedures that the EBP movement focuses on is also apparent.

There are many examples in clinical practice of interventions introduced on assumption of benefit rather than evaluation of impact on a range of outcomes from the perspectives of the relevant stakeholders. In maternity care, universal roll-out of interventions such as routine perineal shaving and enemas at the onset of labor, separation of mothers and babies after birth to prevent infection, and routine use of episiotomy occurred with no supporting evidence that immediate or longer-term outcomes were better—it was assumed that they would be. When these interventions were eventually subjected to rigorous evaluation more often than not there were no differences in outcomes or indications of potential harm (Basevi & Lavender 2008; Carroli & Mignini 2008; Reveiz et al. 2007; Widstrom et al. 1990). The *Term Breech Trial* (Hannah et al. 2000) provides a useful example of why longer-term outcomes from different stakeholders' perspectives need to be considered and evaluated before universal change in practice takes place.

A small proportion of women (around 2–3%) will have a baby which presents at term in a breech presentation and studies which had previously considered which mode of birth was optimal for the baby and for the woman had been inconclusive due to methodological issues and small sample sizes. In certain cases, for example if it was a footling breech or if the baby was large, planned cesarean section (CS) had been considered safer than planned vaginal birth. The Term Breech Trial was designed to provide the ultimate answer to the mode of birth debate, with the proviso that study centers would have clinicians with the expertise to support vaginal breech births. The trial took place in 121 centers in 26 countries and recruited over 2,000 women. Women and their babies were initially followed up to 6 weeks post-birth. Primary study outcomes included perinatal and neonatal mortality or serious neonatal morbidity and maternal mortality or serious maternal morbidity. At 6 weeks, perinatal and neonatal mortality and morbidity were significantly lower among the planned CS group (17 of 1039 [1.6%] versus 52 of 1039 [5.0%]; relative risk 0.33 [95% CI 0.19–0.56]; $p < 0.0001$). There were no differences in any of the maternal outcomes. The trial was stopped early due to a higher event rate than expected. The authors concluded that planned CS was better than planned vaginal birth. Trial results were fast-tracked for publication by *The Lancet* (Hannah et al. 2000) despite need for caution raised by one peer reviewer because of concerns about the impact on practice of differential findings and implications this could have for maternity care in both developed and developing countries (Bewley & Shennan 2007).

Contrary to the usually slow uptake of research findings, in this case, the trial rapidly changed practice in many countries, with planned CS rates rising steeply following publication of the trial (Alexandersson et al. 2005; Carayol et al. 2007; Molkenboer et al. 2003). In England, planned elective CS is now the preferred mode of birth for women with a diagnosed breech baby at term (Department of Health 2008). Debate about the findings of the Term Breech Trial has continued particularly following publication of a two-year planned follow-up of women and babies, which showed no differences in outcomes between the study groups (Whyte et al. 2004). Criticisms of the original trial included lack of adherence to the study protocol, variation in standards of care between trial centers, inadequate methods of fetal assessment, and recruitment of women during active labor when they may not have had a chance to properly consider participation (Glezerman 2006). That women were not supported to birth in upright positions which could have increased the likelihood of a vaginal birth was also criticized (Gyte & Frolich 2001).

Criticisms have been refuted by the trial team who defended their position that this was a peer reviewed trial evaluated in a number of countries and that criticisms in the main reflected the prior beliefs of clinicians (Ross & Hannah 2006).

The worldwide impact of study findings and rapid implementation of its findings into practice has already had an unplanned outcome on the erosion of clinical skills to support vaginal breech birth (Glezerman 2006). As such it is important to consider if immediate and longer-term outcomes and reporting in response to queries raised should have been assessed prior to publication, and if the trial outcomes were the most appropriate for all relevant stakeholders. Practice changed globally based on publication of immediate outcomes, despite criticisms that study results may have been subject to bias due to problems with the trial protocol (Glezerman 2006); however, the longer-term (2 year) outcomes showed no difference (Whyte et al. 2004) which may have been a more reassuring finding for clinicians and for women, posing the issue of which outcomes at which time point should be used to inform practice? In terms of how women were reassured, we would also have to consider the basis for outcomes on which obstetricians defined their expertise in supporting vaginal breech birth and whether outcomes would have differed if midwives had also been involved. The other moot point here is the prior beliefs of those most likely to be implementing change and those likely to be the recipients of the change, and whether an RCT was the most appropriate research method to use given the vagaries of maternity practice context, policy, and culture across the globe (Kotaska 2004). The trial which aimed to provide the definitive answer has changed practice when perhaps it should not have done, given the concerns about the protocol and the presentation and interpretation of outcomes. What is clear is that this trial could never be repeated due to change in routine practice and loss of clinical skills.

## Why do interventions of unproven benefit continue to be implemented?

Although considerable resource has been directed to improving health, implementation of best practice continues to be haphazard. It has been estimated by researchers in The Netherlands and the US that 30–45% of patients do not receive care based on research evidence and that around a quarter of patients receive care which they do not require or which is potentially harmful (McGlynn et al. 2003; Schuster et al. 1998). Audits and national surveys of practice have found that interventions which could improve patient outcomes have not been universally implemented despite evidence of effectiveness—for example, statins in patients who have suffered a cerebral vascular accident (LaRosa et al. 1999) and one-to-one support for women in labor (Redshaw et al. 2007).

One main barrier is that studies rarely address all aspects of a "full-cycle" evidence implementation strategy either because funding is tailored to short-term follow-up only or as evidenced by the Term Breech Trial (Hannah et al. 2000), publication of short-term outcomes inform a change in practice which is difficult to reverse if longer-term outcomes suggest this may not have been necessary. Work to understand how and why the Term Breech Trial changed practice so rapidly when other interventions of proven benefit continue to be implemented piecemeal should be undertaken as this could illustrate how and in what circumstances individual clinicians use evidence, what value they place on the evidence and the influence of their prior beliefs.

Barriers to changing practice in line with evidence of effectiveness can take many forms, including lack of resource for, and poor attention to, dissemination and implementation strategies as illustrated by Grimshaw et al. (2004). Barriers to change could also include lack of necessary equipment or a health providers' reluctance to purchase new equipment due to other competing priorities, use of local pathways or protocols which do not accord with national recommendations, lack of appropriate clinical skills, and low patient adherence with recommended management (Straus et al. 2009). More often than not, challenges to achieving change will occur at different levels and at different points across an organization. Cheater and colleagues (2005) undertook a Cochrane review of tailored interventions to overcome barriers to change and considered effects on professional practice and healthcare outcomes. The objectives of the review were to assess the effectiveness of strategies tailored to address specific, identified barriers to change in professional performance. To meet the objectives, two comparisons were considered: (1) an intervention tailored to address identified barriers to change compared with no intervention or an intervention(s) not tailored to the barriers and (2) an intervention targeted at both individual and social or organizational barriers compared with interventions targeted at only individual barriers.

Fifteen studies were included in the review. The reviewers were unable to identify which barriers were valid, which were the most important, if all barriers had been identified and if they had been addressed by the intervention chosen. The effectiveness of tailored interventions to address barriers to change remains uncertain and further research which also considers process outcomes is required.

As poor interprofessional collaboration and communication could hinder the delivery of health services and patient care, another Cochrane review considered the effects of practice-based interventions on professional practice and healthcare outcomes (Zwarenstein et al. 2009). Five studies were included in the review; data from which suggested that interprofessional interventions could improve healthcare processes and outcomes, but the small number of studies, issues with how collaboration was conceptualized and measured and heterogeneity of interventions and settings meant it was difficult to draw conclusions about the key elements of interprofessional collaboration and its effectiveness.

If we are to ensure approaches to assess the impact and outcomes of EBP are accorded equal priority with the development of methods, theories and frameworks to support the synthesis, critique, and implementation of evidence, it is clear that we need to consider strategic approaches to define what we mean by an "outcome" from the outset of planning an intervention in practice. Davies and Nutley (2008) suggest the following strategic considerations; are we interested in organizational or individual impacts?; who are our key audiences and why do they want information assessing research use and impacts?; will any use and impact assessment be primarily for *learning* (when examinations of process may also need to be emphasized), or will the assessment be primarily to enable *judgments* to be made (requiring examinations of output and outcomes to be emphasized)?

Majumdar (2009) discusses a series of case examples to elicit why some studies are successful in changing practice. Based on the case examples, he found that the studies which were successful had the following in common:

- Addressed a common and clinically important problem,
- Evaluated well-designed interventions,
- Had adequate sample sizes,
- Used reasonable and robust analytic plans,
- Delivered valid results,
- Were published in high-impact general medical journals.

There is a clear need to ensure that if the results of an intervention lead to better outcomes, if they are to be replicated elsewhere *all* components of the intervention must be applied, sufficient details of the intervention have to be available to support those charged with implementation and better descriptions of what a clinically significant outcome would entail would need to be decided at the planning stage.

## The importance of outcomes in policy and politics

Our healthcare systems are subject to the vagaries and fluctuations of political and policy change; a priority for policy in one year may well change the following year. In some cases, change is implemented because of a political motive to garner the populist vote and although this may have an evidence base, the longer-term impacts may not have been fully considered. As referred to earlier with respect to the recommendations of NICE, we also have to be mindful of the powerful role that consumers and industry can play in reversing an unpopular decision about a healthcare intervention, if there are political repercussions for the government of the day.

During recent years we have seen increased reference to the need for evidence-based policy (Department of Health 1999), although many studies continue to assess outcome from an individual perspective (Davies & Nutley 2008). In 1999, a paper from the English Department of Health outlined plans for significant reform of how the UK government would work, which included that policy making would be informed through "better use of evidence and research in policy making and better focus on policies that will deliver long term goals" and would be a continuous learning process (Department of Health 1999, p. 17).

Bodies that fund research, particularly in health and social care are increasingly likely to tailor funding priorities to accord with government policy to increase the usefulness of the research output. This in turn is focussing attention on to how to increase the impact of the research output (Nutley 2003). As Nutley (2003) writes, while there is developing evidence of how to increase impacts of research use on the individual practitioner we know little about the effectiveness of strategies aimed at promoting use of evidence by policy makers. The role of organizations such as the Cochrane and Campbell Collaborations are essential to promote robust research evidence for use by a range of stakeholders, including policy makers. However, active dissemination of findings does not mean that review findings will be reflected in policy directives in the way originally intended by research teams.

What is required now is more methodological work to know when, where, and how to assess the outcomes of use of research. From a policy perspective, dialog is necessary to ascertain if interest is in actual or potential outcomes, given that policy makers may be more interested in immediate recommendations for change due to the political impetus rather than awaiting the longer-term impacts. The outcomes of primary or secondary evidence when used by policy makers are also likely to be subject to integration with other forms of research, knowledge, and expert opinion as well as shifting priorities at government level.

## Conclusion

Throughout the following chapters, authors describe different approaches to capturing data on a range of outcomes. These include specific healthcare service and practice outcomes relevant to the topic of interest, the economic and resource impact of EBP as viewed from the perspective of relevant stakeholders and need to ensure the outcomes a research team consider important are actually a priority from the perspective of the intended target user group. Whichever approach is used, whether quantitative or qualitative, the practical issue of how to evaluate the outcome of EBP in practice has to be addressed. This not only has to reflect an appropriate measure, it also requires consideration of when the outcome should be captured, from whose perspective and implications for future use. We should also pay more attention to process outcomes which could provide information on the influence of context and culture on research use.

## References

Alexandersson, O., Bixo, M., & Hogberg, U. (2005). Evidence-based changes in term breech delivery practice in Sweden. Acta Obstetricia et Gynecologica Scandinavica, 84(6), 584–587.

Basevi, V. & Lavender, T. (2008). Routine perineal shaving on admission in labour. *Cochrane Database of Systematic Reviews*, 1, Art. No. CD001236. doi: 10.1002/14651858.CD001236

Bellomo, R., & Bagshaw, J.M. (2006). Classifying the evidence from clinical trials—The need to consider other dimensions. *Critical Care*, 10:232. doi: 10.1186/cc5045.

Bewley, S. & Shennan, A. (2007). Peer review and the Term Breech Trial. *The Lancet*, 369, 906.

Carayol, M., Blondel, B., Zeitlin, J., Breart, G., & Goffinet, F. (2007). Changes in the rates of caesarean delivery before labour for breech presentation at term in France: 1972–2003. *European Journal of Obstetrics, Gynecology and Reproductive Biology*, 132, 20–26.

Carroli, G. & Mignini, L. (2008). Episiotomy for vaginal birth. *Cochrane Database of Systematic Reviews*, 3, Art. No. CD000081. doi: 10.1002/14651858.CD000081.pub2

Cheater, F., Baker, R., Gillies, C. et al. (2005). Tailored interventions to overcome identified barriers to change: Effects on professional practice and health care outcomes. *Cochrane Database of Systematic Reviews*, 3, Art. No. CD005470. doi: 10.1002/14651858.CD005470

Cochrane, A. (1976). *Effectiveness and Efficiency: Random Reflections on Health Services*. London: The Nuffield Trust.

Davies, H.T.O. & Nutley, S.M. (2008). Learning more about how research-based knowledge gets used. Guidance in the development of new empirical research. William T Grant Foundation, Working Paper.

Department of Health (1999). *Modernising Government. White Paper.* London: The Stationery Office.

Department of Health (2008). *National Maternity Statistics, England 2006–2007*. London: The Information Centre.

Glezerman, M. (2006). Five years to the Term Breech Trial: The rise and fall of a randomized controlled trial. *American Journal of Obstetrics and Gynecology*, 194, 20–25.

Graham, K. & Logan, J. (2004) Using the Ottawa model of research use to implement a skin care programme. *Journal of Nursing Care Quality*, 19(1), 18–24.

Grimshaw, J.M., Thomas, R.E., MacLennan, G. et al. (2004). Effectiveness and efficiency of guideline dissemination and implementation strategies. *Health Technology Assessment*, 8(6).

Gubb, J. (2008). Should patients be able to pay top-up fees to receive the treatment they want? Yes. *British Medical Journal*, 336, 1105.

Guyatt, G., Cook, D., & Haynes, B. (2004). Evidence based medicine has come a long way. *British Medical Journal*, 329, 990–991.

Gyte, G. & Frohlich, J. (2001). Planned caesarean section versus planned vaginal birth for breech presentation at term: A randomised multicentre trial. *MIDIRS Midwifery Digest*, 11, 80–83.

Hannah, M.E., Hannah, W.J., Hewson, S.A. et al. for the Term Breech Trial Collaborative Group (2000). Planned caesarean section versus planned vaginal birth for breech presentation at term: A randomised multicentre trial. *The Lancet*, 356, 1375–1383.

Helfrich, C.D., Li, Y.F., Sharp, N.D., & Sales, A. (2009). Organizational readiness to change assessment (ORCA): Development of an instrument based on the Promoting Action on Research in Health Services (PARIHS) framework. *Implementation Science*, 4, 38. Available online: http://www.implementationscience.com/content/4/1/38.

Hofmeyr, G.J., Neilson, J.P., Alfirevic, A. et al. (2008). *A Cochrane Pocketbook. Pregnancy and Childbirth*. Chichester, England: John Wiley and Son.

Institute of Medicine (2009). Public Meeting 9. The healthcare imperative: Lowering costs and improving outcomes. Available online: http://www. iom.edu/en/Activities/Quality/EBM/2009-MAY-21.aspx.

Kitson, A., Harvey, G., & McCormack, B. (1998). Enabling implementation of evidence-based practice: A conceptual framework. *Quality in Health Care*, 7(3), 149–158.

Kotaska, A. (2004). Inappropriate use of randomised trials to evaluate complex phenomena: Case study of vaginal breech delivery. *British Medical Journal*, 329(7473), 1039–1042.

Lakhani, A., Coles, J., Eayres, D., Spence, C., & Rachet, B. (2005). Creative use of existing clinical and health outcomes data to assess NHS performance in England: Part 1—performance indicators closely linked to clinical care. *British Medical Journal*, 330, 1426–1431.

Lancet (2005). Herceptin and early breast cancer: A moment for caution. *The Lancet*; 336, 1673.

LaRosa, J., He, J., & Vupputuri, S. (1999). Effects of statins on the risk of coronary disease: A meta-analysis of randomized controlled trials. *JAMA*, 282, 2340–2346.

Majumdar, S.R. (2009). Case examples. Chapter 3.8. In: S. Straus, J. Tetroe, & D. Graham (eds) *Knowledge Translation in Health Care: Moving from Evidence to Practice*. Oxford: Blackwell Publishing.

Maynard, A. & Bloor, K. (2009). NICE wobbles. *Journal of Royal Society of Medicine*, 102, 212–213.

Maynard, A., Bloor, K., & Freemantle, N. (2004). Challenges for the National Institute for Clinical Excellence. *British Medical Journal*, 329, 227–229.

McGlynn, E., Asch, S.M., Adams, J. et al. (2003). The quality of health care delivered to adults in the United States. The New England Journal of Medicine, 348, 2635–2645.

Molkenboer, J.F., Bouckaert, P.X., & Roumen, F.J. (2003). Recent trends in breech delivery in The Netherlands. British Journal of Obstetrics and Gynaecology, 110(10), 948–951.

Nutley, S. (2003). Increasing research impact: Early reflections from the ESRC Evidence Network. ESRC UK Centre for Evidence Based Policy and Practice.

Redshaw, M., Rowe, R., Hockley, C., & Brocklehurst, P. (2007). *Recorded Delivery: A National Survey of Women's Experiences of Maternity Care 2006*. Oxford: National Perinatal Epidemiology Unit.

Reveiz, L., Gaitán, H.G., & Cuervo, L.G. (2007). Enemas during labour. *Cochrane Database of Systematic Reviews*, 3, Art. No. CD000330. doi: 10.1002/14651858.CD000330.pub2

Ross, S. & Hannah, M. (2006). Interpretation of the Term Breech Trial findings. *American Journal of Obstetrics and Gynecology*, 195, 1873–1877.

Rycroft-Malone, J. & Bucknall, T. (eds) (2010). *Models and Framework for Implementing Evidence-based Practice: Linking Evidence to Action.* Oxford: Blackwell Publishing Ltd.

Rycroft-Malone R., Seers, K., Titchen, A., Harvey, G., Kitson, A., & McCormack, B. (2004). What counts as evidence in evidence-based practice? *Journal of Advanced Nursing*, 47(1), 81–90.

Sackett, D.L., Rosenberg, W.M.C., Muir Gray, J.A., Haynes, B., & Scott Richardson, W. (1996). Evidence based medicine: What it is and what it isn't. *British Medical Journal*, 312, 71–72.

Schuster, M., McGlynn, E., & Brook, R.H. (1998). How good is the quality of health care in the United States? *Milbank Quarterly*, 76, 517–563.

Sigma Theta Tau International 2005–2007 (2008). Research and Scholarship Advisory Committee Position Statement 2008. *World Views on Evidence Based Nursing*, 5(2), 57–59.

Straus, S.E., Tetroe, J., Graham, I.D., Zwarenstein, M., & Bhattacharyya, O. (2009). Monitoring knowledge use and evaluating outcomes of knowledge use. Chapter 3.6.1. In: S. Straus, J. Tetroe, & I.D. Graham (eds) *Knowledge Translation in Health Care: Moving from Evidence to Practice.* Oxford: Blackwell Publishing.

Titler, M., Steelman, V., Budreau, G., Buckwalter, K., & Goode, C. (2001). The IOWA model of evidence-based practice to promote quality care. *Critical Care Nursing Clinics of North America*, 13(4), 497–509.

Widstrom, A.M., Wahlberg, V., Matthiesen, A.S. et al. (1990) Short-term effects of early suckling and touch of the nipple on maternal behavior. *Early Human Development*, 21, 153–163.

Whyte, H., Hannah, M.E., Saigal, S. et al. (2004). Term breech trial collaborative group: Outcomes of children at 2 years after planned cesarean birth versus planned vaginal birth for breech presentation at term: The international randomized term breech trial. *American Journal of Obstetrics and Gynecology*, 191, 864–871.

Zwarenstein, M., Goldman, J., & Reeves, S. (2009). Interprofessional collaboration: Effects of practice-based interventions on professional practice and healthcare outcomes. *Cochrane Database of Systematic Reviews*, 3, Art. No. CD000072. doi: 10.1002/14651858.CD000072. pub2

# Chapter 2

# Measuring outcomes of evidence-based practice: Distinguishing between knowledge use and its impact

*Ian D. Graham, Debra Bick, Jacqueline Tetroe, Sharon E. Straus, and Margaret B. Harrison*

**Key learning points**

- Consideration and measurement of instrumental, conceptual, and symbolic use of knowledge are important considerations in implementation research.
- Measurement of knowledge use depends on one's definition of knowledge, of knowledge use, and on the perspective of the knowledge user.
- Evaluation of knowledge use can be complex, requiring a multidimensional and iterative approach, focusing at the patient, provider, and system-level outcomes where appropriate.
- A clear starting point in this work is to define the outcomes of interest and to clearly distinguish between consideration and measurement of knowledge use and consideration and measurement of the impacts that knowledge use has on service users/patients, providers, and the health system.

## Introduction

This chapter explores some of the conceptual and methodological issues related to measuring outcomes of evidence-based practice (EBP). EBP is a type of knowledge use, primarily knowledge derived from research. In keeping with many of the planned action models/ theories (Graham et al. 2006), we divide outcomes into two broad categories: knowledge use (use of the evidence underpinning the practice, i.e., behavior change) and its impact (what results from use of that knowledge, i.e., service user/patient outcomes, improved, more efficient and cost effective delivery of care) and discuss some of the conceptual and measurement issues involved. The chapter concludes by considering how measuring outcomes of EBP can demonstrate return on investment in health research.

## Knowledge use

Knowledge use should be monitored during and following efforts to implement EBP (Graham et al 2006). This step is necessary to determine how and to what extent the knowledge has diffused through the target decision-maker groups (Graham et al. 2006). Knowledge uptake is typically complex and examining attitudes and perceptions, and how and where evidence is integrated in decision making influences the success of implementation. It is also an important precursor to other outcome assessment to ensure any positive or negative effects that are attributed to the knowledge use and the main indicator of the success of an intervention to implement EBP. By monitoring knowledge use, identifying when it is sub-optimal and exploring the barriers and supports to knowledge uptake, action can be taken to refine the implementation intervention to overcome the barriers and strengthen the supports. Measuring and attributing knowledge use is still in its infancy within health research. How we proceed to measure knowledge use depends on our definition of knowledge and knowledge use and on the perspective of the knowledge user.

Several models or classifications of knowledge use have been proposed that essentially group knowledge use into three categories: conceptual (indirect), instrumental (direct), and symbolic (persuasive or strategic) use (Beyer & Trice 1982; Dunn 1983; Estabrooks 1999; Larsen 1980; Weiss 1979). Conceptual knowledge use refers to knowledge that has informed or influenced the way users think about issues (i.e., this includes the notion of enlightenment). Measures of conceptual use of knowledge include comprehension, attitudes, or intentions. Instrumental or behavioral knowledge use (Larsen 1980) refers to knowledge that has influenced action or behavior (i.e., direct application of knowledge that influences behavior or practice via incorporation into decision making). Measures of instrumental knowledge use include adherence to guideline recommendations as assessed by process of care indicators. Another form of instrumental knowledge use would include changing policy and procedures, acquiring necessary equipment, or reorganizing staffing or services to enable adherence to EBP (we label this type of knowledge use as enablers of instrumental use). The third category of knowledge use is often referred to as symbolic (persuasive or strategic) knowledge use (Beyer & Trice 1982; Estabrooks 1999; Weiss 1979). Symbolic use involves using research as a political or persuasive tool to legitimize and sustain predetermined positions. It is about using research results to persuade others to support one's views or decisions and thereby may (or may not) lead to either conceptual or instrumental use of that knowledge by others. Symbolic use can be considered as an implementation intervention in some cases. Dunn further categorized knowledge use by describing that it could take place at the individual or collective level (Dunn 1983).

Building on the work of Nutley and colleagues (Nutley et al. 2007), Figure 2.1 depicts our conceptualization of the relationships between knowledge use and its impact. EBP has the potential to impact service user, provider, and system outcomes. Impacts result directly from instrumental knowledge use (applying EBPs) while the effect of conceptual use of EBP is usually through its eventual influence on instrumental use. Knowledge use can be seen as a continuum ranging from conceptual to instrumental use. Any effect of symbolic use of knowledge is mediated through its influence on either conceptual or instrumental use. Enablers of instrumental use create the preconditions that facilitate instrumental use directly (e.g., the adoption of a new policy requires a practice change or incentives are introduced to motivate behavior) and can also influence conceptual use as the individual comes to value the practice change they are required to perform. It should be noted that motivation for behavior change may be intrinsic (as is the case when conceptual use influences instrumental use because the individual believes performing the practice will be beneficial) or extrinsic (as is the case when enablers of instrumental use create the preconditions where behavior change results

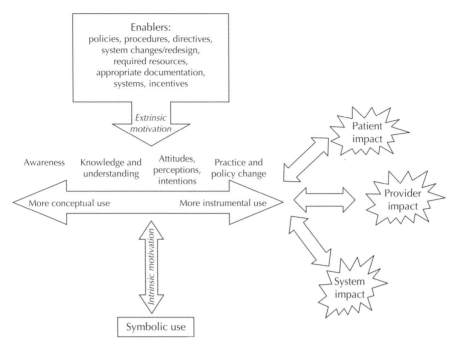

**Figure 2.1** Conceptualization of outcomes of evidence-based practice.

without the individual having to consciously think much about it, e.g., removing a particular test from a test ordering form).

We find it useful to differentiate conceptual, instrumental, and symbolic knowledge use when planning and implementing EBP (Graham et al. 2006). As mentioned above, conceptual use of knowledge implies changes in understanding, attitudes, or intentions. Research could change thinking and be considered in decision making but not result in practice or policy change because the evidence is insufficient; change is not prudent at this time; current practice is close enough, etc. From an EBP perspective, the aim would be to have conceptual knowledge use become the impetus for instrumental use (i.e., a practitioner becomes knowledgeable about a best practice and develops both positive attitudes toward it and intentions to want to do it which in turn motivates action (instrumental use)). Instrumental knowledge use can, however, occur in the absence of conceptual use of that same knowledge, although this is sub-optimal. This is more likely to occur when there are strong incentives to adopt an EBP even when a practitioner may be sceptical or unaware of the underlying evidence for the practice or believe that it will not accrue its expected benefits. In cases such as this, the instrumental use of knowledge is extrinsically, rather than intrinsically, motivated.

An example of conceptual knowledge use comes from a study to increase maternity care nurses' provision of labor support and diminish the use of continuous electronic fetal monitoring. In this study one outcome measure was nurses' self-efficacy for labor support (Davies & Hodnett 2002). Nurses had high levels of self-efficacy related to the desired behavior of labor support, yet this was not correlated with their performance of labor support (instrumental use) (Davies et al. 2002).

Instrumental knowledge use is the concrete application of knowledge in practice that should result in a desired outcome (Graham et al. 2006). An example of instrumental knowledge use is when knowledge that has been transformed into a usable form such as a practice guideline or care pathway is applied to making a specific decision. In the Davies study (Davies et al. 2002), use was measured by the extent to which nurses actually provided labor support and the use of electronic fetal monitoring. Labor support was determined by using a work-sampling approach to measure the proportion of nurses' time spent providing labor support with two independent observers randomly observing nurses during blocks of time and classifying nursing behaviors according to a structured worksheet (Davies et al. 2002). Frequency of use of electronic monitoring was measured by conducting an audit on randomly selected obstetric records. In both cases the measures provided an indication of instrumental use of the recommendations in the fetal health surveillance guideline of interest.

Symbolic knowledge use refers to research being used as a political or persuasive tool to influence others' conceptual or instrumental knowledge use. Knowledge can be used symbolically to, for example, provide a scientific basis for a decision, but it can also be used symbolically to attain specific power or profit goals (i.e., knowledge as ammunition). Another example of symbolic use is for making decisions already taken seem to be evidence based (we call this "decision-based evidence making"). As a positive example, the knowledge of adverse events associated with use of mechanical restraints on agitated inpatients can be used symbolically to persuade the nursing manager on the medical ward to develop a ward protocol about their use. In this example, symbolic knowledge use facilitates understanding by the nurse manager of the issues around mechanical restraints (conceptual use) and prompts her to act (instrumental use).

Further justification for classifying knowledge use into conceptual and instrumental use comes from Grol and Wensing (2005) who reviewed 10 models and theories of stages or steps in the change process originating from different disciplines and revealed how remarkably similar they all were. When these stages are considered in the context of types of knowledge use, all the stages of change models differentiate between conceptual knowledge use—becoming aware of the innovation (e.g., stages labeled awareness, comprehension, seeking information), increasing one's knowledge (stages labeled knowledge, understanding, skills), forming positive attitudes (stages labeled attitude formation, attitude change, agreement, positive attitude), developing intentions to use (stages labeled decision, intention to change), and instrumental use (initial and ongoing use labeled initial implementation, behavior change, change of practice and sustained implementation, consolidation, maintenance of change, routine adherence). Grol and Wensing's own model of the process of change for care providers and teams consists of orientation (promote awareness, stimulate interest), insight (create understanding), acceptance (develop positive attitudes, a motivation for change, create positive intentions or decision to change), change (promote actual adoption into practice), and maintenance (integrate new practice into routines) (Grol & Wensing 2004). All of these models illustrate how knowledge use is conceptualized as a continuum running from awareness, understanding, attitudes, and intentions (conceptual use) through to practice and policy change (instrumental use).

Finally, it should be remembered that with all types of knowledge use, it may be complete or partial. Using the example of practice guideline implementation, the adoption of a guideline with multiple recommendations might result in conceptual use of some recommendations and instrumental use of others. Furthermore, instrumental use of the same guideline might involve intentionally disregarding some recommendations while adhering to others. This can be further complicated when adherence to some recommendations might be complete or partial. In other words, a clinician's approach to recommendations in the same guideline could range from conceptual use of some of them (they understand the recommendation but do not adhere to it), partial instrumental use of some of them (they follow some of the recommendation but not all of it or are not able to follow all of them because of the circumstances of their practice setting) and complete instrumental use of others (they follow the recommendation to the letter).

## Measurement considerations

When thinking about measuring EBP one needs to consider outcomes from several perspectives: definitional, approach to measurement, and selection of measures and tools. The operational definition of the outcome is a first step. This involves determining whether you are interested in measuring knowledge use (and within this broad concept—conceptual, instrumental, or symbolic use) or measuring impact (and at what level) or both. Continuing with the example about the EBP in provision of labor support, the question becomes "how do you wish to operationalize labor support?" What, precisely, do you mean by labor support? Does it include physical, emotional, and spiritual support? How would each of these be defined? Does support for a woman in labor include all support provided during the woman's labor? Is it focused on support provided during certain stages? Is it restricted to health care providers' provision of support? In other words, what exactly is the outcome to be measured?

Measurement of outcomes can be direct or indirect. Direct measures would be ones where the outcome can be directly observed or measured, such as would be the case by observation of the provision of labor support (either by an independent third party, her partner or care provider) or test scores about midwives' or nurses' knowledge about how to provide labor support. Indirect or surrogate measures are ones that only report on the outcome such as documentation in charts of the provision of labor support or its impact on the woman. Measures can also be subjective or objective. Subjective reports such as those based on self-reports by clinicians, women or their partners about the labor support provided often suffer from recall bias. Measures often considered more objective in nature (i.e., less susceptible to recall bias) would include observation and those derived from administrative databases of health records (e.g., the existence of a fetal monitoring strip in the health record indicating (EFM) electronic fetal monitoring). However, measures derived from documents are only as reliable as the quality and thoroughness of the original documentation. Indeed, clinicians may actually be engaged in EBP but not documenting it—for example postnatal records used in some English and Welsh maternity units may be decades old and not revised in line with recent National Institute for Health and Clinical Excellence (NICE) guidance to inform the content of postnatal care (NICE 2006). Methods for collecting outcome measures typically include audit, surveys, interviews, and observation.

Selection of outcome measures should be guided by considerations such as scientific merit and pragmatic issues such as resource requirements to collect the data as well as the potential burden of administration. Issues related to scientific merit require assessment of the available measures as to their reliability, validity, and clinical sensitivity. Meaningful and sensitive measurement requires purposeful consideration of these factors in consultation with the stakeholders in the context of the project or study. The next sections consider issues around the measurement of knowledge use and its impact.

## Measuring knowledge use

As has been suggested, knowledge use is a continuous and complex process that can manifest itself over several events (Rich 1991) rather than a single discrete event occurring at one point in time. Evaluating knowledge use can therefore be complex requiring a multidimensional, iterative, and systematic approach (Sudsawada 2007). Fortunately, there are some tools for assessing knowledge use. Dunn completed an inventory of tools available for conducting research on knowledge use (Dunn 1983). He identified 65 strategies to study knowledge use and categorized them into naturalistic observation, content analysis, and questionnaires and interviews (Dunn 1983). He also identified several scales for assessing knowledge use but found that most had unknown or unreported validity and reliability. Examples of questionnaires available to measure knowledge use include the Evaluation Utilization Scale (Johnson 1980) and Brett's Nursing Practice Questionnaire (Brett 1987). This latter questionnaire focuses primarily on the stages of adoption as outlined by Rogers (Rogers 2003) including awareness, persuasion, decision, and implementation. Estabrooks developed a scale using four questions to measure overall research utilization, direct research utilization (instrumental use), indirect research utilization (conceptual use), and persuasive research utilization (symbolic use) (Estabrooks 1999). Skinner has developed a tool for measuring knowledge exchange outcomes that is undergoing pilot testing (Skinner 2007). This tool consists of two categories: reach (the extent to which best practices are known to potential users, i.e., conceptual use) and uptake (behavioral efforts to use best practices, i.e., instrumental use).

There are a numerous other measures of knowledge use that focus on the multiple decisions required for knowledge use and view the process as a continuum occurring over time. These measures include Halls levels of use scale (Hall et al. 1975) (non-use, orientation (initial formation), preparation (to use), mechanical use, routine, refinement, integration, and renewal), the Peltz and Horsley research utilization index (Peltz & Horsley 1981), the Larson information utilization scale (considered or rejected, nothing done, under consideration, steps toward implementation, partially implemented, implemented as presented, implemented, and adapted) (Larson 1982), and the Knott and Wildavsky stages of research utilization (Knott & Wildavsky 1980). Landry and colleagues have validated this latter scale which includes six stages: reception, cognition, discussion, reference, effort and influence, and implementation (Landry et al. 2001). Landry and colleagues also developed another similar scale to measure knowledge use by policy makers (Landry et al. 2003). Moersch has modified Hall's levels to provide guidance for determining the extent of implementation using seven levels: non-use, awareness, exploration, infusion, integration, expansion, and refinement (Moersch 1995). Champion and Leach developed a knowledge utilization scale that assesses four sets of items: attitudes toward research, availability or access of research, use of research in practice, and support to use research (Champion & Leach 1989).

Most frequently, knowledge utilization tools measure instrumental knowledge use (Estabrooks et al. 2003). In systematic reviews synthesizing the results of studies of effectiveness of interventions to influence the uptake of practice guidelines (Grimshaw et al. 2004; Harrison et al. 2010), measures of instrumental knowledge use (i.e., guideline adherence) are included in upward of 89% of practice guideline implementation studies in medicine, nursing, and allied health professionals included in these reviews (Hakkennes & Green 2006; see Chapter 10).

These measures, however, often rely on self-report and are subject to recall bias. For example, an exploratory case study investigated call center nurses' sustained use of a decision support protocol (Stacey et al. 2006b); participating nurses were surveyed about whether they used the decision support tool in practice. Eleven of 25 respondents stated that they had used the tool and 22 of 25 said they would use it in the future. The authors identified potential limitations to this study including recall bias and a short follow-up period (1 month) without repeated observation (Stacey et al. 2006b). In a more valid assessment of instrumental knowledge use, participants also underwent a quality assessment of their coaching skills during simulated calls (observation of the practitioner–patient encounter) (Stacey et al. 2006a). Assessing instrumental knowledge use can also be done by measuring adherence to recommendations or quality indicators using administrative databases or chart audits. Another way to measure instrumental knowledge use can involve observing service user–clinician encounters and addressing the extent to which the EBPs are used. Asking service users about their health care encounter, which has all the limitations of self-report, is another means of assessing EBP.

Conceptual knowledge use can be measured by tests of knowledge/understanding (e.g., the extent to which clinicians acquire the knowledge and skills taught during training sessions) which is why surveys of attitudes and intentions (e.g., measures of attitudes toward a specific practice, perceptions of self-efficacy performing the practice, or intentions to perform them) are common outcome measures in implementation studies or studies of EBP (Godin et al. 2008). For example, in a randomized controlled trial of an intervention to implement evidence-based patient decision support in a nurse call center, part of the intervention included nurses taking a 3-hour online tutorial (Stacey et al. 2006a). Incorporated into the tutorial was a knowledge test to determine whether the nurses had acquired the relevant knowledge and skills to be able to provide decision support. Around 50% of guideline implementation studies in nursing and allied health professions included measures of conceptual knowledge use compared with less than 20% in medicine (Hakkennes & Green 2006; see Chapter 10).

In addition to considering the type of knowledge use, we should also consider who we want to use the knowledge (i.e., the public or service users, health care professionals, managers/administrators, policy makers). Different target audiences may require different strategies for monitoring knowledge use. For example, when the target is policy makers, a decision to adopt or endorse a particular practice guideline for their jurisdiction enables instrumental use. Assessing the use of knowledge by policy makers may require strategies such as interviews and document analysis (Hanney et al. 2002). When assessing knowledge use by clinicians, we could consider measuring awareness of the existence of guideline recommendations, knowledge of the content of the recommendations and actual application of guideline recommendations.

When implementing EBP, it is also important to consider the degree of knowledge use that we are aiming for. This should be based on discussions with relevant stakeholders including consideration of what is acceptable and feasible and whether a ceiling effect may exist (Straus et al. 2009). If the level of knowledge use is found to be adequate, strategies for monitoring sustained knowledge use should be considered. If the level of knowledge use is less than expected or desired, it may be useful to reassess barriers to knowledge use. Target decision makers could be asked about their intention to use the knowledge. This exploration may uncover new barriers. In the case study of the use of decision support for a nurse call center, a survey of the nurses identified that use of the decision support tool might be facilitated through its integration in the call center database, incorporating decision support training for staff, and informing the public of this service.

## Evaluating the impact of knowledge use

When considering the implementation of EBP, assessing level of knowledge use is important but the bottom line would always be important service user/patient or clinical, provider, and system outcomes. We should not lose sight of the fact that the ultimate goals of EBP are improved health status and quality of care.

Evaluation of impact should start with formulating the question of interest. We find using the PICO framework to be useful for this task (Straus et al. 2009). Using this framework, the "P" refers to the population of interest which could be the public, health care providers, or policy makers. The "I" refers to the implementation/KT intervention which was implemented and which might be compared to another group ("C"). The "O" refers to the outcome of interest which in this situation refers to health, provider or organizational outcomes.

The value of considering the impacts of research utilization in terms of patient, provider, and system or organization outcomes have been discussed elsewhere (Graham and Logan 2004; Logan and Graham 1998). In a systematic review of methods used to measure change in outcomes following an implementation or knowledge translation intervention, Hakkennes and Green (2006) grouped measures into three main categories which we have modified to focus on impact of knowledge use. They are as follows:

(1) service user/patient or clinical level,
  – measures of an actual change in health status such as mortality, morbidity, signs and symptoms, functional status, quality of life, and adverse events,
  – other measures of impact on the service user/patient unrelated to health status such as service user/patient satisfaction,
(2) health care provider level,
  – measures of provider satisfaction,
(3) system or organizational level,
  – measures of change in the health care system (e.g., wait time, length of stay, health care visits, readmissions) or expenditures.

Donabedian's well-known framework separates quality of care into structure, process, and outcome (Donabedian 1988). It can be used to categorize quality indicators and to frame outcomes of both knowledge use and the impact of knowledge use. Structural indicators focus on organizational aspects of service provision which could be analogous to enablers of instrumental knowledge use (e.g., organizational adoption or endorsement of a practice guideline, purchasing equipment practitioners need if they are to be able to adhere to guideline recommendation). Process indicators focus on care delivered to service users and include the communication of evidence to service users and caregivers. These indicators are analogous to instrumental knowledge use. Donabedian's outcome indicators refer to the primary goal of improving service user/patient health outcomes.

For example, if we want to look at the issue of prophylaxis against deep vien thrombosis (DVT) in patients admitted to the intensive care unit, structural measures would include the availability of (DVT) deep vein thrombosis prophylaxis strategies at the institution (enabling instrumental knowledge use). Process measures include prescription of DVT prophylaxis strategies such as heparin in the critical care unit (instrumental knowledge use). Outcome measures would include prevalence of DVT in these patients.

Impact measures are used less frequently than instrumental use outcomes. In the systematic reviews of guideline implementation, of the included studies 65–67% of the studies in nursing and allied health professions respectively included measures of impact compared with 53% of studies in medicine (see Chapter 10). Of guideline implementation studies in medicine, just over 20% included measures of service user/patient health status while under 40% included measures of system impact (Hakkennes & Green 2006).

Table 2.1 describes examples of measures of knowledge use and impact, how they map on to Donabedian's framework, strategies for data collection and possible sources of data. One still needs to decide, however, when to measure knowledge use and when to measure the impact of knowledge use. In cases where the implementation intervention targets a behavior for which there is a strong evidence of benefit, it may be appropriate to measure the outcomes of the intervention only in terms of whether the behavior has occurred (instrumental knowledge) rather than whether a change in service user health status outcomes has occurred (Hakkennes & Green 2006). For example, Ciachini and colleagues recently completed a study of a strategy to implement the Osteoporosis Canada guidelines in a northern Ontario community setting (Straus et al. 2009). The primary outcome of this randomized trial was appropriate use of osteoporosis medications (instrumental knowledge) rather than service user fractures (clinical outcome). They felt that there was sufficient evidence in support of use of osteoporosis medication to prevent fragility fractures that they did not need to measure fractures as the primary outcome. In cases such as this study, outcome measurement at the service user level could be prohibitively expensive, but failure to do so can beg the question of whether or not the intervention improves relevant clinical outcomes.

## Measuring outcomes of EBP and return on investment

Considerable national investments are made in health research with the expectation that when the resulting research findings are applied they will translate into improved prevention and effective treatments of disease and improved population health. Increasingly, governments and funders of health research have begun to show interest in how best to capture the returns on their national investments in health research (Panel on Return on Investment in Health Research

**Table 2.1** Measures of knowledge use and impact

| Construct | Donabedian's construct | Description | Examples of measures | Strategy for data collection | Source of data |
|---|---|---|---|---|---|
| *Knowledge use* | | | | | |
| • Conceptual (service user/patient or provider) | Process | Changes in knowledge levels, understanding, attitudes, intentions | Knowledge; attitudes; intentions to adopt practice | Self-report | Questionnaires, interviews with service users/patients or providers |
| • Instrumental (service user/patient or provider) | Process | Changes in behavior or practice | Adherence to recommendations (e.g., adoption of a new nursing practice or abandonment of existing practice; change in prescribing or test ordering) | Audit, observation, self-report | Administrative database or clinical database, observations of service user/patient–provider encounters, Questionnaires, interviews with patients about provider behavior, questionnaires, interviews with providers |
| • Enablers of instrumental use | Structure | Changes required to enable changes in behavior | Organizational endorsement of guideline recommendations, purchasing of required equipment, changes in policies and procedures (records and forms) | Self-report, document analysis | Interviews, documents |

*(Continued)*

**Table 2.1** (*Continued*)

| Construct | Donabedian's construct | Description | Examples of measures | Strategy for data collection | Source of data |
|---|---|---|---|---|---|
| *Impact* | | | | | |
| • Service user/ patient impact | Outcome | Impact on service users/ patients of using/applying the knowledge | Health status (morbidity or mortality, signs, symptoms, pain, depression); health-related quality of life; function<br><br>Satisfaction with care | Audit, self-report | Administrative database, clinical database, questionnaires, interviews |
| • Provider impact | Outcome | Impact on providers of using/applying the knowledge | Satisfaction with practice; time taken to do new practice | Self-report, observation, | Questionnaires, interviews |
| • System/ Organization impact | Outcome | Impact on the health system of using/applying the knowledge | Length of stay; wait times, readmissions; expenditures and resource use; hospitalizations | Audit, self-report | Administrative database, clinical database, questionnaires, interviews with service users/ patients or providers |

2009). Given that the EBP movement is one important mechanism for increasing the application of research findings by clinicians, it may be useful to consider its fit to frameworks for measuring the impacts of investments in health research.

Beginning in 2005 the Canadian Institutes of Health Research (CIHR), Canada's premier health research funding agency, began work developing a framework and indicators to measure the impacts of health research (Bernstein et al. 2007). This framework and categories to measure impact were adapted from the payback framework developed by Buxton and Hanney (1994). Evolving over time, the impact categories consist of: advancing knowledge, research capacity, informing decision making, health benefits, and economic benefits. In the interim, the Canadian Academy of Health Sciences (CAHS) was commissioned by 26 health research funders (including CIHR) and health professional associations to review existing frameworks, propose a "best framework" and menu of metrics by which to measure return on investment in health research (Panel on Return on Investment in Health Research 2009).

Validating CIHR's impact framework and extending it, the CAHS Return of Investment (ROI) framework proposed the following impact categories and subcategories: advancing knowledge, building capacity, informing decision making (health related, research related, health products industry, general public), health impacts (health status, determinants of health, health care system), and broad economic and social impacts (research activity, commercialization, health benefit, well-being, social benefits). While the first two categories (advancing knowledge and building capacity) are not directly related to our discussion of outcome measures of EBP, the remaining three categories share similarities with our categorization of knowledge use and impacts. The CAHS impact category of *informing decision making* encompass our categories of conceptual and instrumental knowledge use while the CAHS categories of *health impacts* and *broader economic and social impacts* generally map on to our categories of service user/patient, provider, and system impacts. The CAHS ROI framework may therefore be useful for measuring the ROI related to knowledge use and impact of EBP.

## Conclusion

Measuring outcomes of EBP is complex because EBP itself is complex. However, conceptual frameworks of the process of knowledge use can be used to guide the measurement of some of the outcomes of EBP. The starting point is clearly defining the outcomes of interest and distinguishing between knowledge use (the conceptual, instrumental or symbolic use of the knowledge underlying EBP) and the impacts of EBP on service users/patients, providers, and the system. A multitude of strategies can be used to collect data on outcomes ranging from self-report by service users/patients and providers to audit of health records and documents to observation of health encounters between service users/patients and providers. Each strategy has strengths and limitations that should be carefully considered.

Use of a combination of strategies, resources allowing, would enable triangulation of data to improve face and content validity. The complexity and nascency of measuring EBP is a challenge for applied researchers trying to demonstrate the impact of their work. However, by working within a framework (such as the CAHS ROI framework) they can focus their evaluation on specific outcomes with the understanding that these outcomes are situated within a larger (unmeasured) context.

# References

Bernstein, A., Hicks, V., Borbey, P., Campbell, T., McAuley, L., & Graham, I.D. (2007). A framework to measure the impacts of investments in health research. In: *Science, Technology and Innovation Indicators in a Changing World*, Paris: OECD, pp. 231–249.

Beyer, J.M. & Trice, H.M. (1982). The utilization process: A conceptual framework and synthesis of empirical findings, *Administrative Science Quarterly*, 27(591), 622.

Brett, J.L. (1987). Use of nursing practice research findings, *Nursing Research*, 36(344), 9.

Buxton, M. & Hanney, S. (1994). Assessing Payback from Department of Health Research & Development: Preliminary Report, Health Economics Research Group (HERG), Brunel University, Uxbridge, UK, p. 19.

Champion, V.L. & Leach, A. (1989). Variables related to research utilization in nursing: An empirical investigation, *Journal of Advanced Nursing*, 14, 705–710.

Davies, B.L. & Hodnett, E. (2002). Labour support: Nurses' self-efficacy and views about factors influencing implementation, *Journal of Obstetric, Gynecology and Neonatal Nursing*, Jan–Feb.(31), 1–48.

Davies, B.L., Hodnett, E., Hannah, M., O'Brien-Pallas, L., Pringle, D., & Wells, G. (2002). Fetal health surveillance: A community-wide approach versus a tailored intervention for implementation of a clinical practice guideline, *Canadian Medical Association Journal*, 167(5), 469–474.

Donabedian, A. (1988). The quality of care. How can it be assessed?, *Journal of the American Medical Association*, 260, 1743–1748.

Dunn, W.N. (1983). Measuring knowledge use, *Knowledge: Creation, Diffusion, Utilization*, 5(120), 33.

Estabrooks, C. (1999). The conceptual structure of research utilization, *Research in Nursing Health*, 22(203), 16.

Estabrooks, C., Floyd, J., Scott-Findlay, S. et al. (2003). Individual determinants of research utilization: A systematic review, *Journal of Advanced Nursing*, 43(506), 20.

Godin, G., Belanger-Gravel, A., Eccles, M., & Grimshaw, J. (2008). Healthcare professionals' intentions and behaviors: A systematic review of studies based on social cognitive theories, *Implementation Science*, July(3), 36.

Graham, I.D. & Logan, J. (2004). Innovations in knowledge transfer and continuity of care, *Canadian Journal of Nursing Research*, 36(2), 89–103.

Graham, I.D., Logan, J., Harrison, M.B. et al. (2006). Lost in knowledge translation: Time for a map?, *Journal of Continuing Education of the Health Professions*, 26(13), 13–24.

Grimshaw, J., Thomas, R.E., MacLennan, G. et al. (2004). Effectiveness and efficiency of guideline dissemination and implementation strategies, *Health Technology Assessment*, 8(6).

Grol, R. & Wensing, M. (2004). What drives change? Barriers to and incentives for achieving evidence-based practice, *Medical Journal of Australia*, 180(Suppl. 6), S57–S60.

Grol, R. & Wensing, M. (2005). Effective implementation: A model. In: R. Grol, M. Wensign, & M. Eccles (eds) *Improving Patient Care*. Edinburgh: Elsevier, pp. 41–57.

Hakkennes, S. & Green, S. (2006). Measures for assessing practice change in medical practitioners, *Implementation Science*, 1, 29.

Hall, B., Loucks, S., Rutherford, W., & Newlove, B. (1975). Levels of use of the innovation: A framework for analyzing innovation adoption, *Journal of Teacher Education*, 26(1), 52–56.

Hanney, S.R., Gonzalez-Block, M.A., Buxton, M.J., & Kogan, M. (2002). The utilization of health research in policy-making: Concepts, examples and methods of assessment, *Health Research Policy and Systems*, 1, 2.

Harrison, M.B., Graham, I.D., Godfrey, C.M., Medves, J.M., & Tranmer, J. (2010). Guideline dissemination and implementation strategies for nursing and allied health professions, *Cochrane Library* (under review).

Johnson, K. (1980). Stimulating evaluation use by integrating academia and practice, *Knowledge*, 2(237), 62.

Knott, J. & Wildavsky, A. (1980). If diffusion is the solution: what is the problem?, *Knowledge: Creation, Diffusion, Utilization*, 1(4), 537–578.

Landry, R., Amara, N., & Lamari, M. (2001). Climbing the ladder of research utilization. Evidence from social science research, *Science Communication*, 22, 396–422.

Landry, R., Lamari, M., & Amara, N. (2003). The extent and determinants of the utilization of university research in government agencies, *Public Administration Review*, 63, 192–204.

Larsen, J. (1980). Knowledge utilization. What is it?, *Knowledge: Creation, Diffusion, Utilization*, 1, 412–442.

Larson, J.K. (1982). *Information Utilization and Non-utilization*. Palo Alto, CA: American Institutes for Research in the Behavioral Sciences.

Logan, J. & Graham, I.D. (1998). Toward a comprehensive interdisciplinary model of health care research use, *Science Communication*, 20(2), 227–247.

Moersch, C. (1995). Level of technology implementation (LoTi): Framework for measuring classroom technology use, *Education Technology*, Nov., 40–42.

National Institute for Health and Clinical Excellence (NICE) (2006). *Routine Postnatal Care of Women and Their Babies. NICE Clinical Guideline 37. National Collaborating Centre for Primary Care*. London: RCOG Press.

Nutley, S., Walter, I., & Davies, H. (2007). What works to promote evidence-based practice – cross sector experiences. In: *Implementation and Translational Research*. Stockholm, Oct. 14–16.

Panel on Return on Investment in Health Research (2009). *Making an Impact. A Preferred Framework and Indicators to Measure Returns on Investment in Health Research*. Ottawa, ON: Canadian Academy of Health Sciences.

Peltz, D.C. & Horsley, J.A. (1981). Measuring utilization of nursing research. In: J.A. Ciarlo (ed.) *Utilization Evaluation: Concepts and Measurement Techniques*. Beverley Hills, CA: Sage, pp. 125–149.

Rich, R.F. (1991). Knowledge creation, diffusion, and utilization: Perspectives of the founding editor of Knowledge, *Knowledge: Creation, Diffusion, Utilization*, 12, 319–337.

Rogers, E. (2003). *Diffusion of Innovations*, 5th ed. New York, NY: Free Press.

Skinner, K. (2007). Developing a tool to measure knowledge exchange outcomes. *Canadian Journal of Program Evaluation*, 22(1), 49–73.

Stacey, D., O'Connor, A., Graham, I.D., & Pomey, M.P. (2006a). Randomised controlled trial of the effectiveness of an intervention to implement evidence-based patient decision support in a nursing call centre, *Journal of Telemedicine and Telecare*, 12(410), 15.

Stacey, D., Pomey, M.P., O'Connor, A., & Graham, I.D. (2006b). Adoption and sustainability of decision support for patients facing health decisions: An implementation case study in nursing, *Implementation Science*, 1, 17.

Straus, S., Tetroe, J., Graham, I.D., Zwarenstein, M., & Bhattacharyya, O. (2009). Monitoring and evaluating knowledge. In: S. Straus, J. Tetroe, & I.D. Graham (eds) *Knowledge Translation in Health Care*. Oxford: Wiley-Blackwell, pp. 151–159.

Sudsawada, P. (2007). *Knowledge Translation. Introduction to Models, Strategies, and Measures*. Austin, TX: Southwest Educational Development Laboratory, National Center for the Dissemination of Disability Research.

Weiss, C.H. (1979). The many meanings of research utilization. *Public Administration Review*, Sept., 426–431.

# Chapter 3

# Models and approaches to inform the impacts of implementation of evidence-based practice

*Joyce Wilkinson, Neil Johnson, and Peter Wimpenny*

---

**Key learning points**

- Review some key terms related to models of implementation
- Be introduced to a typology of models of implementation based on work of Nutley et al. (2007)
- Through this typology, be able to discuss the focus of a variety of extant models of implementation and their contribution to impact of evidence on practice
- Conclude on the use of the typology, the fit of models and the nature of future use in practice.

---

## Introduction

This chapter will focus on developing an understanding of the utility and purpose of implementation models, which are described in more detail in Book 1 of this series (Rycroft-Malone & Bucknall, in press). A model typology will be used to assist this understanding drawn from empirical work on research use by Nutley et al. (2007). Such a typology enables us to classify implementation models and begin to focus on the different kinds of impacts that may be identified as a result of their application. Published examples are discussed in illustrating the differing foci of implementation models and the impacts identified from their use.

This chapter concludes by summarizing and highlighting the main aspects of the types of models and the impacts that these might inform, and reflects on the implications for their selection and use in practice.

However, firstly it is useful to describe some of the key terms that will be used throughout the chapter and for which there may be a myriad of interpretations.

## Models

Many terms are used to describe what we have included in this chapter as models and we have sought to be inclusive, rather than exclude on the grounds of title. Instead, we have included anything which had as its aim a means of guiding, explicating, exploring, or representing in diagrammatic format, the evidence or research into practice process. These have variously been presented or described as models, strategies, approaches, diagrams, and frameworks and include those which are conceptual, theoretical, and empirically based. We have called them models for the purposes of this chapter.

## Evidence-based practice

For ease of use, we will use the term "evidence" as an all-encompassing one, to include research, routine monitoring of data, experience, and expert opinion, all the while trying to focus on the process and impacts, rather than get drawn into wider debates about the nature of evidence. That said we also recognize that the nature of evidence and practitioners' views of that, does, in itself, have an impact on the ways in which they engage with the evidence-into-practice process.

Likewise, the term "evidence-based" practice (EBP) leaves scope for varying interpretations, with the terms "evidence-informed" becoming more prominent as a means of reflecting the numerous ways in which evidence has the potential to influence practice, beyond being an obvious "base" on which practice changes or develops. Indeed, the different ways in which evidence can impact on practitioners is explored in more detail, later in this chapter, but cannot always be traced to an evidence-base or attributed to specific types or pieces of evidence. However, once again, rather than get sidetracked on semantic debates, we will use the term that is most familiar that of EBP.

## Implementation and utilization

We view implementation as a process, not an event, through which evidence, practitioners and the work environment (and this could include patients also) are prepared to carry out some change in practice. We view this as a change management process that also involves evaluation and readjustment to allow for ongoing use of evidence which may not always be explicit or observable.

## Impact

Dictionary definitions of impact suggest force and change, often hinting at some magnitude as we would associate with the impact of, for example, two cars colliding. However, we believe that impact from the use of evidence can be viewed as "difference"—the difference that using evidence has made for patients, practitioners, and local and national health-care organizations. These may be of some magnitude and of some reach or influence, but others may be much more subtle and not readily identified, even by practitioners themselves. Seeing impact as difference embraces a spectrum of impacts and therefore allows us the greatest potential to identify and highlight the numerous ways in which evidence can make a difference in practice. From this standpoint the models and impacts that we explore in this chapter can be seen to demonstrate or have the potential to demonstrate a broad range of measurable and less easily measurable impacts.

## A model typology

The model typology (Figure 3.1) has been adapted from empirical work, which focused originally on the ways in which evidence was

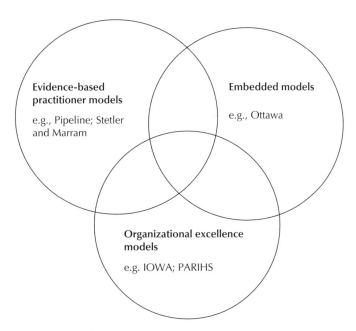

**Figure 3.1** Model typology.

used in social care (Walter et al. 2004) and wider empirical and conceptual work relating to research use across the public sector, including health care, through the Research Unit for Research Utilization at the University of St Andrews. The typology enables us to identify some main features of any model within three broad types.

A typology can be helpful in seeking to illuminate different models and their impact in the world of EBP as well as providing a more discerning analysis of the elements potentially enabling impacts to occur.

There are challenges in doing this. The boundaries where the three model types overlap create some blurring and it may be that there are wider areas of overlap than those shown. Another challenge is the lack of detail for some models which make the classification into a particular type difficult. For example, the IOWA model (Titler et al. 2001) instructs *institute change in practice* but does not provide detail as to how this should or could take place and as a result, it is more difficult, for example, to determine where it should sit. One further limitation of this typology is that despite the overall aim of models being to focus on guiding, testing, tracing or assisting the implementation of evidence into practice, detailed examination is not undertaken and if it is, there is no consensus on what should be examined. This makes any comparison difficult. An additional confounding factor is the lack of detail provided in published examples in relation to outcomes as they often focus much more on process. That said there is recognition that process impacts are still of importance and may be of equal significance in improving patient outcomes and in our understanding of the relationships between the factors contributing to the implementation of evidence-into-practice.

The features of each of the three model types are described below in Boxes 3.1–3.3.

These three different model types with their different approaches and foci will, we contend, determine different types of approaches to evidence use and therefore impacts for practitioners, practice, patients, and health-care organizations could also be different. Each of the model types will now be examined in more detail with illustrations from papers where a specific model has been used.

## Evidence-based practitioner models

This model type reflects some of the earlier thinking in the evidence utilization field, in which the focus was predominantly on the ways in which individual practitioners could and should access evidence, appraise it, and if relevant, then use it in their practice.

---

**Box 3.1 The evidence-based practitioner models**

The main features or underlying principle or assumptions of the models are as follows.

- It is the role and responsibility of the individual practitioner to keep abreast of evidence and ensure that it is used to inform or act as a basis for day-to-day practice.
- This process is a linear one, which involves the practitioner accessing, appraising, and applying evidence to practice.
- Practitioners have high levels of professional autonomy to change practice to reflect evidence.
- Professional education, development, and training are important in enabling practitioners to use evidence in practice.

*Source*: Adapted from Walter et al. (2004) and Nutley et al. (2007).

---

---

**Box 3.2 The embedded evidence models**

The main features or underlying principles or assumptions of the models are as follows.

- Evidence use is achieved by a process of embedding evidence into the systems and processes of care provision, such as policies, standards, guidelines, protocols, procedures, and tools.
- Responsibility for ensuring evidence use lies with policy makers, guideline developers, and service delivery managers.
- The use of evidence is both a linear and an instrumental process: evidence is directly translated into practice change.
- Funding, performance management, and regulatory regimes are used to encourage the use of evidence-based guidance and tools.

*Source*: Adapted from Walter et al. (2004) and Nutley et al. (2007).

---

**Box 3.3 The organizational excellence models**

The main features or underlying principles or assumptions of the models are as follows.

- The key to successful evidence use rests with health-care organizations: their leadership, management, and organization.
- Evidence use is supported by developing an organizational culture that is "evidence-minded."
- There is local adaptation of evidence and ongoing learning within organizations in an attempt to use local data as evidence for improvement of care.
- Partnerships with local universities and other intermediary organizations are fostered to facilitate both the creation and use of evidence for practice.

*Source*: Adapted from Walter et al. (2004) and Nutley et al. (2007).

---

Despite the problems that began to emerge with this approach, for example, those identified by Hunt in her seminal paper of 1981, (such as practitioners' lack of autonomy to change practice and lack of practitioner skills to read and appraise research) this is still a model that is widely considered to be the dominant means of getting evidence into practice although literature suggests that there may be an emergent sum of evidence to counter such a view (Rycroft-Malone et al. 2004). Rogers (1983) argued that in many instances individual adoption of new innovations (or in this case evidence) cannot occur unless organizational adoption occurs first. However, more recently Wilkinson (2008) has shown that nurse managers still believe that the full responsibility for EBP lies with individual staff and although some barriers to this are recognized, such as varying individual skills and ability, these are not considered to be such that nurses' responsibilities for evidence use by this approach are negated.

The dominant aspect of this model type is the evidence content and the process of appraising and applying it to practice. For example, Heneghan et al. (2007) use the Pipeline model (Glasziou 2005; Glasziou & Haynes 2005) to consider the use of hypertension guidelines in a family doctor practice. The acceptability of the evidence to practitioners (and patients) is paramount, but ultimately adherence to the evidence is the "step" that is viewed as having the most impact in practice. It is a linear approach to evidence use that assumes that practitioners will have the knowledge, authority, and autonomy to make evidence-informed changes to their own practice.

This model reflects the understanding that the experiential knowledge of practitioners will be used to consider evidence and then make decisions about its appropriateness and subsequent use in practice. In the same way, the views of patients may also be taken into account, but there are difficulties relating to the precedence given to any particular aspect of this process and the primacy of some evidence (such as research) over other types (such as patient choice) and how these can be given equal footing. Thompson et al. (2001) have shown that nurses value the experience and opinion of others over published research and this was also borne out in other work (Wilkinson 2008). These highlight the difficulties of trying to use practitioner models in assessing impact when the types of evidence favored by practitioners can vary significantly and the decision-making processes that surround the choice of evidence and the accompanying processes that see it implemented or used in practice are so difficult to understand or articulate.

The evidence-based practitioner models also assume or reflect a belief that practitioners have, by dint of their professional status or specific job role, a level of autonomy over practice that will allow them to use evidence after they have accessed and appraised it. Heneghan et al. (2007) report on the changes to hypertension management by family doctors. Glaszious' Pipeline model (2005) may be more applicable to doctors who are possessed of greater levels of autonomy over practice than other professional groups (Dopson & Fitzgerald 2005). The Pipeline model (Glasziou 2005) as illustrated in Heneghan and colleague's (2007) paper, ends with adherence to evidence, but impacts or outcomes beyond this are not made explicit. Despite this, other impacts might be recognized at different stages of the model which may be considered to move the model to a more organizational type (Wimpenny et al. 2008) or from models that have the individual practitioner as the main focus.

The Stetler–Marram (1976) model also illustrates some of the difficulty in employing a practitioner-based model. The use of the Stetler model by McGuire (1990) highlights the lack of research appraisal skills in staff suggesting that implementation may be about more than just autonomy but also about knowledge and understanding of research and evidence in a variety of formats. However, subsequent use of the model for implementation may have been enhanced by the earlier experience and an increase in appraisal skills. Other models, such as the Ottawa Model of Research Utilization (Graham & Logan 2004), do identify the evidence itself as a factor in implementation but the model is focused more distinctively on the broader organizational structures and processes that may limit or assist the evidence into practice. While this may highlight issues of autonomy, reports of use do not identify this as a significant factor (Ellis et al. 2007; Graham & Logan 2004; Hogan & Logan 2004; Logan et al. 1999) suggesting the focus is not on the individual practitioner.

The above highlight the limitations of this model type, that is evidence use is viewed as a largely linear and uncomplicated process, which fails to take account of the numerous "barriers." Studies undertaken now over two decades and in many countries and practice settings (e.g., Bryar et al. 2003; Dunn et al. 1998; Nilsson Kajermo et al. 1998; Oranta et al. 2002; Parahoo, 2000; Parahoo & McCaughan 2001; Restas 2000) show consistently that many practitioners *do not* believe that they have the necessary autonomy, authority, and skills to make changes to practice. This is not to say that some practitioners do not manage to make changes to practice that reflect evidence, but they are not the majority and they often work in roles that "give" them greater clarity and explicit autonomy than most practitioners.

If we try to consider the types of impacts that this model type might facilitate, the issues of access to evidence, skills to appraise and apply to practice, and the ability to take account of different sources of evidence and the need for explicit autonomy to be able to make changes to practice, several points begin to emerge. There are a number of factors that may inhibit any potential impact, such as individual practitioners' skills and abilities, as well as organizational factors, such as local communication and the limits of authority and autonomy to make changes to practice, for either groups of practitioners or individuals. While this may limit the direct instrumental use of evidence in practice, the impact of these models may be seen in other ways (Box 3.4), which may, in time (although this is speculation or hope, rather than any certainty at this point) generally lead to greater use of evidence in practice.

Beyond those practitioners who have or are able to develop the skills that are necessary prerequisites, the impacts are likely to be negligible as the hurdles or barriers are just too great for individual practitioners to overcome. Even where they do have the autonomy (such as medical practitioners) there is often an underlying concern

---

**Box 3.4 Potential impacts from evidence-based practitioner models**

The potential impacts from using the evidence-based practitioner models may be:

- Increased knowledge and skills of individual practitioners for accessing, appraising, understanding, and using evidence to answer specific clinical problems.
- Increased awareness of different types of evidence and their applicability or appropriateness to practice for individuals (conceptual rather than instrumental use).
- Increased confidence in considering the need to change practice to better reflect evidence which may lead to changes to job role, such as a promoted post or involvement in evidence use projects at local or national level. These impacts could be considered as professional development for individuals.
- Impacts on wider teams, units or organization are likely to be limited, but will depend to a greater or lesser extent on the sphere of influence of the individual(s) involved.
- Increased networking or collaborations linked to evidence use may develop (Walter et al. 2005) and links to or development of continuing professional development or continuing education initiatives may take place as the result of these models having an impact for individuals, but also beyond the individual practitioner.

that evidence for the effectiveness of EBP is lacking (Miles et al. 2003) and a review of initiatives in social care (Walter et al. 2004) also suggest that individual skills and autonomy for evidence use are not the whole story in identifying impacts from evidence use in practice. Overall organizational encouragement or professional direction (such as that from the UK Nursing and Midwifery Council) to use evidence in practice, in the way suggested by this model type, does not clearly translate into use of evidence that can be readily identified or traced. The impact on patients from these models is likely to be very difficult indeed to attribute to the models without wider organizational structures and cultures that favor, enable, and support evidence use. Furthermore, this model type does not reflect the sources of knowledge for practice favored by nurses (Thompson et al. 2001; Wilkinson 2008) and any attempts to identify and trace evidence use processes would need to take account of the potential of the multiple sources of evidence available to practitioners and the ways in which these might be synthesized to inform practice. Many of these aspects of evidence-into-practice process, although known of, are as yet poorly understood.

The potential impacts seen in Box 3.4 are offered as examples and are not viewed as an exhaustive list of every impact that might occur through the use of this model type. There are some impacts that may be conspicuous by their absence, such as those relating to improved patient outcomes, greater patient satisfaction or major changes to the ways in which care is provided. That is not to say that these types of impacts could not occur, but that it is less likely, and these types of impacts may be more readily identified through the use of other models. The potential of this model type also relies on the ability of practitioners to "unlearn" (Rushmer & Davies, 2004) routines and practices, as well as their ability to discover and use new evidence and ways of working. The use of practitioner-only-focused models might well be considered the dominant mode of evidence into practice for professionals, but their use, and therefore impact, is more likely to be haphazard and opportunistic and thus their potential impacts difficult to identify and measure.

## Embedded evidence models

The embedded model type focuses on an approach to getting evidence used in practice without (necessarily) clearly identifying it as evidence. Those using evidence rarely engage directly with it and it is presented for use in practice in the form of guidelines, policies, procedures, protocols, or standards for care. Its provenance may not be known to the end user. There is an implicit understanding that these evidence products will be linked in with the tacit knowledge of practitioners, and will "make sense" to them.

The links in the embedded models are not initially between evidence and practitioners, but between evidence networks, policy makers, national agencies (such as the Scottish Intercollegiate Guideline Network, The National Institute for Health and Clinical Excellence or NHS Quality Improvement Scotland) and to organizational networks within health care that serve as intermediaries between these and practitioners. The responsibility for changing practice, or incorporating evidence, lies beyond health-care organizations and individual practitioners. Their respective roles are to communicate the evidence through internal networks and to facilitate their use and ensure adherence to the evidence content. Once again, it is largely a linear process, often from the top down, with the main focus on achieving instrumental use, with less focus on practitioner autonomy or authority to change practice. In fact, in contrast to the evidence-based practitioner models, this may actually be a barrier to the use of embedded models (Nutley et al. 2007; Walter et al. 2004). Use of these evidence products in practice may be demanded by the nature of the product (e.g., a policy would "have to" be adhered to) or controlled by the availability of specific equipment or resources (Wilkinson, 2008). It may also relate to the topic or subject area (Wimpenny & van Zelm 2007). In addition, the use of these products may be monitored and reported on in a routine manner through national schemes. Failure to adhere might be identified at local level through critical incident review or reporting, although the impact of not using an evidence-based product that should have been in use is acknowledged as being a somewhat negative example.

These models often involve different levels within organizations rather than focusing on ward level, since embedding of evidence also requires engagement at meso and macro levels, particularly important for effective dissemination as a necessary pre-condition for implementation processes. If the incorporation of evidence into products such as local guidelines or protocols for care takes place through organizational structures, such as shared governance arrangements, this will still require wider levels of engagement than that of individual wards/units or practitioners to be effective. The Ottawa Model of Research Use (OMRU) provides examples of attempts to embed evidence. The earliest of these reports is Logan et al. (1999) where pressure ulcer guidelines are implemented in a range of clinical settings. It is interesting to note that the "turmoil" of restructuring within the organization was an identified barrier to implementation and highlights the likelihood that there will never be ideal organizational conditions for implementation. While embedded evidence model types will seek to take account of contextual barriers and facilitators these will always be present. Graham and Logan (2004) in a later paper describe the use of the OMRU to introduce a skincare program in five different organizational units, again reflecting a more strategic level approach to embedding evidence for practice across a health-care organization. Although Graham and Logan (2004) report "significant outcomes" from this approach, these are not stated or explicated in the paper.

In a different environment, Ellis et al. (2007) report on the use of the Ottawa model to guide the application of pain measurement tools for children. Again this is at unit level rather than focusing on individual practitioners and illustrates the use of OMRU as predominantly an embedding model type. However, Elllis et al. (2007) do report on the outcomes of use of pain scales (increased use, rather than widespread adoption), but the extent to which this leads to better outcomes or beneficial impact on patients is implicit, rather than clearly stated. Could the model have been used more effectively to assist in embedding evidence, through the use of a pain chart, into practice? If adherence was less than optimal or expected, why might this have been so and was this related to the choice or use of the model?

The impact of embedded evidence might be identified through local audits or the development of local protocols arising from national policies or directives, such as those used for the audit of water quality for dialysis patients, the use of nurse-led thrombolysis protocols or the supply of pressure-relieving mattresses (Wilkinson, 2008). These examples had each developed from national initiatives or directives, the latter, arising from the directive to rationalize the use of resources in one Scottish Health Board as a means of saving money but not compromising on care provision. The adoption of a local tool to assess pressure risk (but based on wider evidence) was underpinned by a Health Board wide protocol that determined the need for hiring-in expensive pressure-relieving mattresses and if appropriate, ensuring that these would be used for the minimum of time and returned promptly to minimize costs. However, none of these examples appeared to be guided or underpinned by the use of an explicit model such as OMRU, which has evaluation of patient, practitioner and health-care system outcomes as an integral part of the model.

These latter examples show that embedding evidence has the potential to demonstrate impact not only at the patient level, but also at meso and macro levels within health-care organizations. However, the example provided relating to the use of pressure mattresses may highlight the potential conflicts between "the evidence" and the patient's choice. The patient may well prefer to spend longer on the supremely comfortable hired in mattress; however, "the evidence" may show that once the patient is able to turn themselves in bed or mobilize independently, there is no clinical benefit (i.e., improved outcome) to continuing to use the expensive mattress. In these situations practitioners may choose to ignore the protocol to reflect "patient choice evidence" over that of research and resource minimization.

As the focus of the embedded model appears to be less on the individual practitioner and more on the evidence products as a means to implementation, then the organizational networks and systems to facilitate their route into practice environments will impact on the extent to which they can be of use there. Often within organizations, the focus becomes "stuck" on these networks and evidence fails to complete the journey into practice if one aspect of the network of distribution or dissemination fails. Review of the (former) Clinical Standards Board for Scotland (CSBS) reports into the implementation of clinical governance (Wilkinson 2008; Wilkinson et al. 2004) identified that in many health-care organizations the focus was on developing verbal and written communication networks but not on considering their effectiveness as a means of seeing evidence used in practice. Even where opportunities existed to develop practice at unit or individual level, based on national evidence products, these were missed.

Reports of use of the Stetler model (McGuire 1990; Reedy et al. 1994) highlight this "sticking of evidence" issue in their recognition that the embedding process took significantly longer than they had anticipated. The development of protocols for drug administration was a lengthy process and was further impeded by concerns raised by practitioners as to some aspects of the protocol. Likewise, use of the Stetler (1994) model to improve bereavement care (Hanson &

Ashley 1994) reflected that the evidence-into-practice process took considerably longer than the staff involved had anticipated due to a perceived poor "fit" of evidence to local context and therefore the incorporation of this into local products. However, this latter example illustrates the potential for other impacts or outcomes from the use of this type of model, as it stimulated thinking about inconsistencies in current care provision and as such could be seen to have a conceptual, rather than instrumental impact on care. In addition Hanson and Ashley (1994) report that changes to follow-up practice of the bereaved did take place, but were not based on the evidence reviewed as part of the overall process. This could be viewed as an unintended outcome or impact, but questions remain as to what these changes were based upon, if not evidence and the extent to which the Stetler model assisted such process outcomes?

Although changes to local culture and practice from the use of embedded evidence have been recognized (Wilkinson 2008) this was not by intentional use of a model, nor was it measured in any way, although the impact on patients was seen by practitioners as beneficial. Indeed, in the example identified by Wilkinson (2008) of health-care assistants using a national nursing best-practice statement for the promotion of continence, this resulted from an educational initiative for staff, rather than a specific attempt to promote the use of evidence in practice. This demonstrates that although different models exist, it might be the adoption of other means that have the greater impact on practice. The health-care assistants in this example were unaware that they were using evidence, or promoting the use of evidence by encouraging qualified nurses to follow their lead in managing some evidence-based aspects of care.

The existence of evidence products for embedding is not likely to be enough to have a significant (or even any) impact on practice. There will still be a need for other engagement through, for example, educational and clinical skills development and for favorable organizational contexts (McCormack et al. 2002; Rycroft-Malone et al. 2004) to support their use in practice. The role of monitoring in increasing adherence and identifying positive outcomes for patients through embedded models is not yet known and may not be as straightforward as it would at first appear, as outlined in Chapter 4 of this book. Issues of ownership and the perceived relevance of evidence have the potential to impede embedded models, if the evidence is somehow seen as being disguised to make it more palatable in certain contexts, or if it is presented in candid manner, which might also create tensions around issues of ownership that will influence on the impact of evidence use and cannot be readily addressed by the models.

A summary of the potential impacts from the use of the embedded models is provided in Box 3.5.

## Organizational excellence model types

This model type focuses not on individual practitioners, nor on the embedding of evidence products per se, but on wider aspects of the organizations that provide health care. Within these organizations the focus is on leadership, management, and organization to

---

**Box 3.5  Potential impacts from embedded evidence models**

The potential impacts of the embedded evidence models are as follows.

- Impacts on process, rather than outcome, may be identified.
- "Stronger" evidence may be thought to have a greater impact, through its embedding into guidelines and policies for national and local use, but this is not necessarily the case since there are complexities arising from the judgments about strengths of evidence versus very specific applicability and the organizational contexts into which they are introduced that will affect evidence use.
- The impacts on individual practitioners are likely to be less of a focus in embedded models, with a greater focus on organizations or teams. Practitioners may be unaware of using evidence in practice and therefore measuring their use of evidence by using self-report, may not be a true reflection of actual use of evidence.
- While the focus of embedded models is not on individuals, there may still be a need for provision of education or practice development initiatives to instruct them in the use of new protocols or approaches to care provision, which might have an impact at individual level of themselves.
- The adoption of evidence into policies and guidelines and the provision of these in a local context for staff does not equate to their use. Considering the impact that these models might have needs to take account of this.
- Impacts for patients may reflect their consultation or involvement in the development of evidence products, but not necessarily improved outcomes for them.

provide the ideal and necessary conditions for evidence use. The role and contribution of professional and ancillary staff is recognized, but it is seen within the wider organizational structures and culture that values, promotes, and enables evidence use. While, on the face of it, some of these features may be seen as reflecting aspects of the embedded evidence model, the focus here is different. The organization is not seen as a mere repository of evidence products, produced elsewhere and provided through the organization for use. Instead, the focus in organizational excellence models is on recognizing complexity, rather than simpler linear models of evidence use. Organizational excellence models often reflect the cyclical and complex nature of evidence use processes, rather than viewing them as straightforward linear, unidirectional ones.

The Promoting Action on Research Implementation in Health Services (PARIHS) model (Kitson et al. 1998) illustrates the interaction between different factors influencing evidence-into-practice processes that may be influential (interactions between the evidence, the context, and facilitation). Local experimentation with evidence, evidence products, and evidence-into-practice processes are all encouraged, with variation that reflects differing local circumstances, experiential knowledge, and patient preferences all being acceptable. Quite contrary to the possible individual or top-down approach of the previous two model types (and indeed the ethos of the evidence-into-practice movement in many health-care initiatives) (Wilkinson et al. 2004), organizational excellence models positively encourage bottom-up initiatives, and sharing across and outside the local area as a means of encouraging and spreading the use of evidence in practice, all recognized features of organizational learning (Kelly et al. 2007; Rushmer et al. 2004a–c, 2006, 2007).

The IOWA model (Titler et al. 1994) illustrates other elements of this model type through involvement of higher education institutions, other disciplines, and different levels of management in an attempt to look beyond the health-care organization to improve practice through the use of evidence as a basis for care (Titler et al. 2001). It also recognizes the importance of involving researchers in the implementation process (White et al. 1995), which is increasingly recognized as an important aspect of knowledge translation (Walter et al. 2004).

This organizational excellence type approach encourages and arranges links with evidence production institutions, and sees the value of a co-ordinated approach to also improving the interest and skills of individual practitioners for evidence use, through Continuing Professional Development (CPD) and educational opportunities. Posts that "add value" to both health-care and higher educational institutions, such as joint appointments (lecturer/practitioner posts or researcher/practitioner posts) have the scope to extend networks and improve communication in both organizations. These "boundary spanner" roles (Greenhalgh et al. 2004) are acknowledged as being important in facilitating and supporting evidence use. The PARIHS model (Harvey et al. 2002) acknowledges the role of facilitation as a key factor in evidence implementation processes and while the exact nature of facilitation and locally appointed facilitator roles may vary, they are seen as significant within an organizational excellence model type.

Likewise opportunities to link education and practice or research and practice environments provide scope for the co-production of evidence, an iterative, rather than linear process that reflects aspects of both environments. Seeing the process as a shared endeavor not only values the contribution of both, but also challenges the myth that practice is the passive recipient of knowledge received from higher authorities, thus making it more relevant and reflective of local priorities, values, and culture.

These local networks may have impacts in addition to those on patient care. They link different levels of organizations, as identified by Dontje (2007) in the use of the IOWA model. However, these model types still have the improvement of patient care at their heart as illustrated by the use of the PARIHS model to evaluate care services for the elderly (Conklin & Stolee 2008). This is a more unusual use of a model of this type but identifies the scope for considering outcomes beyond the point of evidence implementation and sustained use in practice. Further examples of the utilization of the PARIHS model are seen in its use to develop systematic and rigorous approaches to the management of postoperative pain (Brown & McCormack 2005). Using the three elements from this model the authors undertook an appraisal of relevant literature leading to evidence-based conclusions and recommendations for future practice and research. Although no empirical "instrumental" impact in patient care is seen from Brown and McCormack's paper there are clear benefits demonstrated in and around the notion of conceptual impact at the levels of values and beliefs within organizations. With a "user-pull" (Landry et al. 2001a,b) mode underpinning organizational excellence models such as the PARIHS model it can be argued that such impacts at conceptual level are central to enabling conditions which are conducive to evidence translation into practice. Further evidence of the use of the PARIHS model in assisting in re-conceptualizing the relationships between the elements causative toward evidence-based nursing and therefore reshaping beliefs, knowledge, and insight (i.e., conceptual impacts) is seen in a numerous papers using this as a guiding framework (Ellis et al. 2005; Doran & Sidani 2006; Kavanagh et al. 2007). Although impacts of this type are helpful (Sudsawad 2007), in acknowledging the complexity and comprehensiveness of the PARIHS model, it does suggest that more empirical studies of the models application (and therefore impact upon patient outcomes) in health-care environments is needed.

The IOWA model explicitly includes measurement and monitoring of impact beyond implementation (i.e., after the introduction and initial utilization of EBP) and is, to some extent, unique in this regard. While OMRU also includes the evaluation of outcomes, IOWA is explicit in relating this to monitoring structure, process and outcomes data. Titler (2007) sees the strengths of this model as being its use of ranges of evidence, foci on implementation and evaluation of impact upon patient care, and the need to embed this evidence into organizational quality improvement and clinical effectiveness initiatives. Taylor-Piliae (1999) reports on the use of the IOWA model to change unit practices for endotracheal suctioning to an evidence-based guideline. The changes to practice remained in place 2 years after their introduction. Of course, this may also reflect features of the practitioner and embedding types of model. The outcomes and impacts were not only related to improved patient care, but also increased staff satisfaction and cost savings, demonstrating the range of impacts possible from the use of a broader organizational excellence model approach. Further evidence of this model's utility in terms of practice change is illustrated by Gordon et al. (2008) where impacts relating to practice standards and staff education were achieved in the area of neonatal umbilical arterial blood sampling. It would appear from published use of the IOWA model that it has potential to act as a vehicle for reappraisal of practice, evidence and guiding implementation rather than a framework for planning change alone.

Additional impacts might also include the creation of new posts or the development of existing services, such as library and information services, which have the potential to have greater impacts for individual staff although their impact on patients may be less tangible.

The organizational excellence model type reflects the complexities of evidence use to a greater extent than other models and they are more likely to focus on developing an understanding of local circumstances and their own organization as a whole, rather than on specific types of evidence or increasing the evidence use skills of individuals. It is clear that this could also apply to the overarching work reported on using the Stetler model (McGuire 1990), whereby the model was selected to operationalize the organizational excellence approach. The refinement of the Stetler model over time (2001) reflects a growing understanding of the need to focus on organizations rather than individuals to facilitate evidence implementation. The use of OMRU model, which facilitated effective group activity within the organization (Graham & Logan 2004), can also be viewed as providing an organizational excellence approach.

That is not to say, however, that within organizations that have adopted the excellence approach, these other issues are not also attended to, but that they are not the main focus of effort to encourage and facilitate evidence use in organizations. The potential impacts of these models are outlined in Box 3.6.

Once again, these are not presented as the sum total of every possible impact from the adoption of organizational excellence model type, but rather as examples of the kinds of ways that this model type might impact on evidence use.

Diffusion of innovations (Rogers 1995) may also be viewed within the organizational excellence type. It has been used as a means of studying the extent of research or evidence use in organizations, for example, a study undertaken by Luckenbill-Brett (1989) focused on the extent of research use and uses Rogers (1983) theory to explain this. She concludes that it highlights the acceptability of a specific innovation (piece of research) and the ability of an organization to disseminate this, but also identifies many other significant factors, such as how an individual nurses' ability to understand or access research has contributed to use. Taylor-Piliae (1998) also uses Rogers' (1995) theory of the diffusion of innovations as a means of stating the specific factors that nurses in the critical care setting must attend to prior to implementing EBP, but the paper does not describe an initiative of this nature "in action." The expected outcomes relate to the improvement of care through the use of evidence as a basis for practice. Dooks (2001) in an exploration

> **Box 3.6 Potential impacts of organizational excellence models**
>
> The potential impacts of the adoption of organizational excellence models may be the following:
>
> - A change to the culture of organizations to one that values, seeks to understand, and improve the use of evidence in practice.
> - The development of new roles and posts to develop and support evidence use across the organization.
> - The creation and/or development of new links to evidence-producing bodies such as higher education institutions or research institutes.
> - The development of leadership and management skills and traits or the harnessing of these as an important aspect of furthering evidence use.
> - The impact on certain clinical conditions may be greater than that on others due to the national focus on those providing access to increased resources, which the organization harnesses. These may result in specific impacts relating to these clinical conditions, rather than reflecting wider evidence use across organizations.
> - In attempting to view evidence use processes in the widest sense, there may be positive impacts on individual practitioners through, for example, improved access to evidence-based resources or greater autonomy to make changes to practice through the support from bottom-up initiatives.

of the diffusion of pain management research into nursing practice conceptualizes the process of implementation using Rogers' diffusion of innovations model and illustrates the models' value through analysis of it's four main elements (innovation, adopter, communication, and social relationships) in identifying the challenges of integrating best evidence into pain management—something again which may have impact at conceptual level for practitioners working in this field, managers and decision makers.

However, Dooks (2001), in citing an earlier study by Ferrell et al. (1993) serves to demonstrate the model's propensity in achieving improvements in pain management in practice through the careful selection of "early adopters" to develop Pain Resource Nurses, which following a 3-month period, demonstrated improvements in nurses attitudes, educational improvements, and an increase in understanding regarding multidisciplinary awareness in pain management in 92% of nurses surveyed: furthermore evaluation data provide evidence that this innovation was adhered to beyond implementation (Dooks 2001). Further evidence of Rogers' model having positive impact on patient care is illustrated in Kovach et al.'s (2008) use of the principles underpinning the model in improving care in patients with dementia. The findings from this study support the model's potential to make positive changes in the standards of care and the performance of health providers.

There are other such approaches to evidence implementation that are flexible and non-standard in application, such as action research (Parahoo 2006). Its format and reach varies considerably from context to context and application to application. As such it is not possible to "fit" it into a specific type of model in our typology. It is suggested that it can be used in relation to evidence use in a number of ways and as a research approach it offers flexibility to reflect local circumstances and arrangements. Does this then offer the best hope for understanding and developing our knowledge of evidence use impact? Pearcey and Draper (1996) took an action research approach to support the development of a protocol for providing pre-operative information for patients, but were unsuccessful in achieving this goal. This would suggest that the flexibility of the approach is not the universal panacea for evidence implementation projects and having some structure or guide of a particular model (Pipeline, OMRU, Stetler, PARIHS, IOWA) can be helpful. However, on a similar theme, Jester and Williams (1999) used an action research approach to review pre-operative fasting times, consult the literature, devise a standardized approach, and implement the same, with reported significant benefits for patients, through the elimination of prolonged fasting times. As an approach it reflects some aspects of each of the areas of the typology, as it may place a greater emphasis on individual practitioners, embedding of evidence or an organizational excellence approach or embrace all over the course of its use in any specific setting.

In terms of seeking to overcome the complexities of social systems in health care, action research is based upon a fairly programmatic approach of problem identification/diagnosing followed by action (e.g., changes to practice protocols, staff education) and evaluation of impact. In recognizing that the success of any implementation strategy will effect change in either the structure or function of this social system (an analogy drawn from Rogers' definition of diffusion and social change; Rogers 1995), albeit with limited generalizability, McElroy and Sheppard (1999) demonstrate this premise in a participatory action research study reviewing the assessment and management of self-harming patients in an accident and emergency department. It is clear from this study that action research has the potential to affect impacts at individual, departmental, and organizational levels. Process impacts, identified earlier in this chapter, are also identifiable from published projects adopting an action research approach (Lee 2009).

Tranmer et al. (1995) report on the use of an amalgamation of models (Roberts & Burke 1989; Stetler & Marram 1976) underpinned by the CURN (Horsley et al. 1978) model to undertake a research utilization project in a neonatal unit. As a result it appears to be a hybrid of our typology, with different stages of their project reflecting each of the three model types. Their first stage was on up-skilling individual practitioners to enable them to access and appraise research (the individual practitioner model). Then they went on to support nurses to identify areas for practice change and to develop *developmentally sensitive care principles* (embedded evidence models) for care delivery and finally to support their application to practice and to assess their effectiveness in improving patient outcomes. Although the whole health-care organization was not engaged in the way that the organizational excellence models reflect, there were some aspects of these models, such as the alliance that developed between the local nursing research institution and the strengthening of these links to enhance both research and practice, which were evident. The development of a research facilitator post in their project is one aspect of the organization excellence models. In addition, there was a clear recognition of the need to engage nursing management in the project to ensure their support in terms of access to resources and finance. Impacts and outcomes were recognized at all stages of the project, such as an increase in individual nurses' research critique skills, the adoption of new care practices, increased job satisfaction for nurses, and improved teamwork through the development and expression of shared values across the neonatal unit. Notably, impacts or improved patient outcomes are implicit, but presumed, through the reported dissemination of *developmentally sensitive care principles*, such as dimming of the unit lights and the adoption of new positions for babies in incubators, thought (by the staff) to be more *developmentally sensitive*. The use of these measures by staff other than those specifically involved in the project was seen as a significant impact, particularly in terms of standardizing improved practice. This example is unique in terms of its adoption of a hybrid model to guide the research project, but is a useful illustration of the scope of impacts that can be recognized through the use of models and this typology.

## Conclusion

As described in the above example, some models do not fit into one or other type and exhibit features of two or more. As with all aspects of researching or using evidence into practice, this reflects the complexity of the process, the multiple factors involved and our own, still incomplete, understanding of the ways these impact on each other and therefore on impacts that might result from the use of any particular type, or model.

As Nutley et al. (2007) reflect, our own knowledge of these approaches is still such that we are unable to determine whether those models that exhibit shared features (of the typology) are likely to be more effective than those that sit squarely in one type rather than another. The boundaries between the types should be blurred and some models sit nearer to the boundaries than others, reflecting their greater (or lesser) focus on specific characteristics. Likewise, it is impossible to say whether any one type of model is better suited to identifying and measuring impact than any other, only that they focus on different characteristics and will therefore illuminate different types of impact. It is also impossible to state with any confidence whether a combination of all characteristics of all the types of models would lead to the greatest impact identification, or if indeed it would be possible to amalgamate the models. While there may be synergies between them, there are also areas of tension and the different foci of each approach would make this difficult to do, since they are, in some aspects, fundamentally so different.

None of the models illustrated within the typology should be seen as superior to any other, they are all just different, and their use may be restricted until we have a better understanding of why some models have more appeal than others to any individual or organization. By providing examples of the use of some of the models from the literature, we have aimed to provide an insight into some of the ways in which different impacts can be identified and that all impacts are not necessarily related to improved patient outcomes. We have deliberately avoided flagging up the potential negative impacts of some of the types of models, due largely to the limits of space, but also in an effort to remain focused and positive in a area of health care where views that are often diametrically opposed (e.g., evidence use is the universal panacea (Trinder & Reynolds 2000); to evidence use holds no benefit for patients (Miles et al. 2003)) and in trying to understand evidence-into-practice processes we fare no better, often shifting between views that it is a linear process dependent on individual practitioners possessing the essential knowledge and skills and one that sees the whole complex nature of evidence use as multifactorial and nigh on impossible to fathom, let alone tackle. However, we do acknowledge that there may be negative or unintended impacts of the use of any or all of these types of models at macro, meso or micro levels. The different types of models appear to us to provide a framework for those who are seeking to put evidence into practice. This framework may vary from a more conceptual guide (DOI, Action Research, PARIHS) to one which provides more functional guidance (Stetler, IOWA) and those which have components of both (OMRU, Pipeline).

Ultimately, we have sought to show that there are a range of potential impacts from the use of evidence-into-practice models and processes. Whether these models are selected by those who are seeking to develop or improve these impacts is not known. In reality, from what we know about the organizational and practice environments in health care, their use is more likely to be opportunistic, haphazard, or pure chance, yet they still have something to offer those who would seek to better understand the identification of the impact of evidence use in practice and should be viewed in this light. Even if they are not used to guide or inform evidence use processes with impact or outcomes in mind, they have scope as conceptual or theoretical tools to identify processes that have been used and aid the identification, and possibly measurement of impact.

## Acknowledgment

We would like to acknowledge the support of Dr Isobel Walter, University of St Andrews, to the early development of our thinking around implementation, models, and outcomes.

# References

Brown, D. & McCormack, B. (2005). Developing postoperative pain management: Utilising the Promoting Action on Research Implementation in Health Services (PARIHS) framework. *Worldviews on Evidence-based Nursing*, 2(3), 131–141.

Bryar, R.M., Closs, S.T., Baum, G. et al. (2003). The Yorkshire BARRIERS project: A diagnostic analysis of the barriers to research utilization. *International Journal of Nursing Studies*, 40, 73–84.

Conklin, J. & Stolee, P. (2008). A model for evaluating knowledge exchange in a network exchange context. *Canadian Journal of Nursing Research*, 40(2), 116–124.

Dontje, K. (2007). Evidence-based practice: Understanding the process. Implementing evidence-based nursing: The IOWA model. *Advanced Nursing Practice eJournal*, 7(4). Available online: http://www.medscape.com/viewarticle/567786 (last accessed June 29, 2009).

Dooks, P. (2001). Diffusion of pain management research into nursing practice. *Cancer Nursing*, 24(2), 99–103.

Dopson, S. & Fitzgerald, L. (2005). *Knowledge to Action? Evidence-based Health Care in Context*. Oxford: Oxford University Press.

Doran, D. & Sidani, S. (2006). Outcomes-focused knowledge translation: A framework for knowledge translation and patient outcomes improvement. *Worldviews on Evidence-based Nursing*, 4(1), 3–13.

Dunn, V., Crichton, N., Roe, B., Seers, K., & Williams, K. (1998). Using research for practice: A UK experience of the BARRIERS scale. *Journal of Advanced Nursing*, 27, 1203–1210.

Ellis, I., Howard, P., Larson, A., & Roberston, J. (2005). From workshop to work practice: An exploration of context and facilitation in the development of evidence-based practice. *Worldviews on Evidence-based Nursing*, 2(2), 84–93.

Ellis, J.A., McLeary, L., Blouin, R. et al. (2007). Implementing best practice pain management in a pediatric hospital. *Journal of Science of Pain Nursing*, 12(4), 264–277.

Ferrell, B., Grant, M., Ritchley, K., Ropchan, R., & Rivca, M. (1993). The pain resource nurse program: A unique approach to pain management. *Journal of Pain Symptom Management*, 8(8), 549–556.

Glasziou, P. (2005). The paths from research to improved health outcomes [Editorial]. *American College of Physicians Journal Club*, 142(4), A8–A10.

Glasziou, P. & Haynes, B. (2005). The paths from research to improved health outcomes. *Evidence-based Nursing*, 8, 36–38.

Gordon, M., Bartruff, L., Gordon, S., Lofgren, M., & Widness, J. (2008). How fast is too fast? A practice change in umbilical arterial catheter sampling using the IOWA model for evidence-based practice. *Advances in Neonatal Care*, 8(4), 198–207.

Graham, K. & Logan, J. (2004). Using the Ottawa model of research use to implement a skin care programme. *Journal of Nursing Care Quality*, 19(1), 18–24.

Greenhalgh, T., Robert, R., Bate, P., Kyriakiddu, O., McFarlane, F., & Peacock, R. (2004). *How to Spread Good Ideas: A Systematic Literature Review of the Literature and Diffusion, Dissemination and Sustainability of Innovations in Health Service Delivery and Organisation*. London: NCCSDO.

Hanson, J.L. & Ashley, B. (1994). Advanced practice nurses' application of the Stetler model for research utilization: Improving bereavement care. *Oncology Nursing Forum*, 21(4), 720–724.

Harvey, G., Loftus-Hills, A., Rycroft-Malone, J. et al. (2002). Getting evidence into practice: The role and function of facilitation. *Journal of Advanced Nursing*, 37(6), 577–588.

Heneghan, C., Perera, R., Mant, D., & Glasziou, P. (2007). Hypertension guideline recommendations in general practice: Awareness, agreement, adoption, and adherence. *British Journal of General Practice*, 57(545), 948–952.

Hogan, D. & Logan, J. (2004). The Ottawa model of research use. A guide to innovation in the NICU. *Clinical Nurse Specialist*, 18(5), 255–261.

Horsley, J.A., Crane, J., & Bingle, J.D. (1978). Research utilization as an organizational process. *Journal of Nursing Administration*, 8, 4–6.

Hunt, J. (1981). Indicators for nursing practice: The use of research findings. *Journal of Advanced Nursing*, 6, 184–189.

Jester, R. & Williams, S. (1999). Pre-operative fasting: putting research into practice. *Nursing Standard*, 13(39), 33–35.

Kavanagh, T., Watt-Watson, J., & Stevens, B. (2007). An examination of the factor enabling successful implementation of evidence-based acute pain practices into pediatric nursing. *Children's Health Care*, 36(3), 303–321.

Kelly, D., Lough, M., Rushmer, R.K., Wilkinson, J.E., Greig, G.J., & Davies, H.T.O. (2007). Delivering feedback on learning organization characteristics—using a Learning Practice Inventory. *Journal of Evaluation in Clinical Practice*, 13(5), 734–740.

Kitson, A., Harvey, G., & McCormack, B. (1998). Enabling implementation of evidence-based practice: A conceptual framework. *Quality in Health Care*, 7(3), 149–158.

Kovach, C.R., Morgan, S., Noonan, P.E., & Brondino, M. (2008). Using principles of diffusion of innovation to improve nursing home care. *Journal of Nursing Care Quality*, 23(2), 132–139.

Landry, R., Amara, N., & Lamari, M. (2001a). Utilization of social science research knowledge in Canada. *Research Policy*, 30, 333–349.

Landry, R., Amara, N., & Lamari, M. (2001b). Climbing the ladder of research utilization. Evidence from social science research. *Science Communication*, 22(4), 396–422.

Lee, N.J. (2009). Using group reflection in an action research study. *Nurse Researcher*, 16(2), 30–42.

Logan, J., Harrison, M.G., Graham, I.D., Dunn, K., & Bissonnette, J. (1999). Evidence-based pressure ulcer practice: The Ottawa model of research use. *Canadian Journal of Nursing Research*, 31(1), 37–52.

Luckenbill-Brett, J.L. (1989). Organisational integrative mechanisms and adoption of innovations by nurses. *Nursing Research*, 38, 105–110.

McCormack, B., Kitson, A., Harvey, G., Rycroft-Malone, J., Titchen, A., & Seers, K. (2002). Getting evidence into practice: The meaning of "context". *Journal of Advanced Nursing*, 38(1), 94–104.

McElroy, A. & Sheppard, G. (1999). The assessment and management of self-harming patients in an accident and emergency department: An action research project. *Journal of Clinical Nursing*, 8(1), 66–72.

McGuire, J. (1990). Putting research findings into practice: Research utilization as an aspect of the management of change. *Journal of Advanced Nursing*, 15, 614–620.

Miles, A., Grey, J.E., Polychronis, A., Price, N., & Melchiorri, C. (2003). Current thinking in the evidence-based health care debate. *Journal of Evaluation in Clinical Practice*, 9(2), 95–109.

Nilsson Kajermo, K., Nordstrom, G., Krusbrant, A., & Bjorvell, H. (1998). Barriers to and facilitators of research utilization as perceived by a group of registered nurses in Sweden. *Journal of Advanced Nursing*, 27, 798–807.

Nutley, S.M., Walter, I., & Davies, H.T.O. (2007). *Using Evidence. How Research Can Inform Public Services*. Bristol: The Policy Press.

Oranta, O., Routasalo, P., & Hupu, M. (2002). Barriers and facilitators of research utilization among Finnish registered nurses. *Journal of Clinical Nursing*, 11, 205–213.

Parahoo, K. (2000). Barriers to and facilitators of, research utilization among nurses in Northern Ireland. *Journal of Advanced Nursing*, 31(1), 89–98.

Parahoo, K. (2006). *Nursing Research. Principles, Process and Issues*, 2nd ed. Basingstoke: Palgrave Macmillan.

Parahoo, K. & McCaughan, E.M. (2001). Research utilization among medical and surgical nurses: A comparison of their self reports and perceptions of barriers and facilitators. *Journal of Nursing Management*, 9, 21–30.

Pearcey, P. & Draper, P. (1996). Using the diffusion of innovations model to influence practice: A case study. *Journal of Advanced Nursing*, 23, 714–721.

Reedy, A.M., Shivnan, J.C., Hason, J.L., Haisfield, M.E., & Gregory, R.E. (1994). The clinical application of research utilization: Amphotericin B. *Oncology Nursing Forum*, 21(4), 715–719.

Restas, A. (2000). Barriers to using research evidence in nursing practice. *Journal of Advanced Nursing*, 31(3), 599–606.

Roberts, C. & Burke, S. (1989). *Nursing Research: A Qualitative and Quantitative Approach*. Boston: Jones & Bartlett.

Rogers, E.M. (1983). *Diffusion of Innovations*. New York: Free Press.

Rogers, E.M. (1995). *Diffusion of Innovations*. New York: Free Press.

Rushmer, R. & Davies, H.T.O. (2004). Unlearning in health care. *Quality and Safety in Health Care*, 13(Suppl. II), ii10–ii15.

Rushmer, R., Kelly, D., Lough, M., Wilkinson, J.E., & Davies, H.T.O. (2004a). Introducing the learning practice-I, the characteristics of the learning organisation in Primary Care. *Journal of Evaluation in Clinical Practice*, 10(3), 375–386.

Rushmer, R., Kelly, D., Lough, M., Wilkinson, J.E., & Davies, H.T.O. (2004b). Introducing the learning practice-II, becoming a learning practice. *Journal of Evaluation in Clinical Practice*, 10(3), 387–398.

Rushmer, R., Kelly, D., Lough, M., Wilkinson, J.E., & Davies, H.T.O. (2004c). Introducing the learning practice-III, leadership, empowerment, protected time and reflective practice as core contextual conditions. *Journal of Evaluation in Clinical Practice*, 10(3), 399–405.

Rushmer, R., Kelly, D., Lough, M., Wilkinson, J.E., Greig, G.J, & Davies, H.T.O. (2006). Organizational learning: The learning practice: diagnosing and developing learning practices in the UK; the learning practice inventory. In: A.L. Casebeer, A. Harrison, & A.L. Mark (eds) *Innovations in Health Care: A Reality Check*. Basingstoke: Palgrave Macmillan.

Rushmer, R., Kelly, D., Lough, M., Wilkinson, J.E., Grieg, G.J. & Davies, H.T.O. (2007). The learning practice inventory: Diagnosing and developing learning practices in the UK. *Journal of Evaluation in Clinical Practice*, 13(2), 206–211.

Rycroft-Malone, J., Harvey, G., Seers, K., Kitson, A., McCormack, B., & Titchen, A. (2004). An exploration of the factors that influence the implementation of evidence into practice. *Journal of Clinical Nursing*, 13, 913–924.

Stetler, C. (1994). Refinement of the Stetler/Marram model for application of research findings to practice. *Nursing Outlook*, 42, 15–25.

Stetler, C. (2001). Updating the Stetler model of research utilization to facilitate evidence-based practice. *Nursing Outlook*, 49, 272–279.

Stetler, C. & Marram, G. (1976). Evaluating research findings for the applicability in practice. *Nursing Outlook*, 24(9), 59–563.

Sudsawad, P. (2007). *Knowledge Translation: Introduction to Models, Strategies and Measures*. Austin, TX: The National Center for the Dissemination of Disability Research. Available online: http://www.ncddr.org/kt/products/ktintro/ktintro.pdf (last accessed January 16, 2009).

Taylor-Piliae, R.E. (1998). Establishing evidence-based practice: Issues and implications in critical care nursing. *Intensive and Critical Care Nursing*, 14, 30–37.

Taylor-Piliae, R.E. (1999). Utilization of the IOWA model in establishing evidence-based practice. *Intensive and Critical Care Nursing*, 15, 357–362.

Titler, M. (2007). Translating research into practice. Models for changing clinician behaviour. *American Journal of Nursing*, 107(6), 26–33.

Titler, M.G., Kleiber, C., Steelman, V. et al. (1994). Infusing research into practice to promote quality care. *Nursing Research*, 43(5), 307–313.

Titler, M., Steelman, V., Budreau, G., Buckwalter, K ., & Goode, C. (2001). The IOWA model of evidence-based practice to promote quality care. *Critical Care Nursing Clinics of North America*, 13(4), 497–509.

Thompson, C., McCaughan, D., Cullum, N., Sheldon, T., Mulhall, A., & Thompson, D. (2001). Research information in nurses' clinical decision making what is useful? *Journal of Advanced Nursing*, 36(3), 376–388.

Tranmer, J., Kisilevsky, B., & Muir, D. (1995). A nursing research utilization strategy for staff nurses in the acute care setting. *Journal of Nursing Administration*, 25(4), 21–29.

Trinder, L. & Reynolds, S. (2000). *Evidence-Based Practice. A Critical Appraisal*. Oxford: Blackwell Science.

Walter, I., Nutley, S., Percy-Smith, J., McNeish, D., & Frost, S. (2004). *Improving the Use of Research in Social Care Practice*, Social Care Institute for Excellence (SCIE). Bristol: The Policy Press.

Walter, I., Nutley, S., & Davies, H. (2005). What works to promote evidence-based practice? A cross sector review. *Evidence & Policy, A Journal of Research Debate and Evidence*, 1(3), 335–363.

White, J.M., Leske, J.S., & Pearcey, J.M. (1995). Models and process of research utilization. *Nursing Clinics of North America*, 30(3), 409–420.

Wilkinson, J.E. (2008). *Managing to Implement Evidence-Based Practice in Nursing? An Exploration and Explanation of the Roles of Nurse Managers in Evidence-Based Practice Implementation*. Doctoral thesis, University of St Andrews. Available online: http://research-repository. st-andrews.ac.uk/handle/100023/560.

Wilkinson, J.E., Rushmer, R.K., & Davies, H.T.O. (2004). Clinical governance and the learning organisation. *Journal of Nursing Management*, 12, 105–113.

Wimpenny, P. & van Zelm, R. (2007). Appraising and comparing pressure ulcer guidelines. *Worldviews on Evidence-Based Nursing*, 4(1), 40–50.

Wimpenny, P., Johnson, N., Walter, I., & Wilkinson, J.E. (2008). Tracing and identifying the impact of evidence—the use of a modified pipeline model. *Worldviews on Evidence-Based Nursing*, 5(1), 3–12.

# Chapter 4

# An outcomes framework for knowledge translation

*Diane M. Doran*

---

**Key learning points**

- Outcomes-focused knowledge translation provides an approach to knowledge translation that links patient outcomes, measurement, and feedback with research evidence and patient preferences, to encourage evidence-based practice (EBP).
- One mechanism by which outcomes feedback is expected to improve EBP and treatment outcomes involves critical reflection about what is working and what is not working in patient care. A second mechanism by which outcomes feedback is expected to improve treatment outcomes may involve improved communication between the clinician and patient.
- Intuitive reasoning, a relatively automatic form of reasoning, which can stem either from instinctual cognitive processes or from highly practiced, over-learned behavior, is subject to a well-known range of biases and contextual errors. The goal of outcomes-focused knowledge translation is to stimulate rational deliberative reasoning about the patient's response to health-care intervention and about the most appropriate patient-care interventions.
- Outcomes-focused knowledge translation could be used in combination with other validated approaches for knowledge translation that include attention to the context of care.

## Introduction

This chapter describes the conceptual framework for knowledge translation that is known as outcomes-focused knowledge translation (Doran & Sidani 2007). Knowledge translation is defined as "the exchange, synthesis and ethically sound application of researcher findings within a complex system of relationships among researchers and knowledge users" (Canadian Institutes of Health Research, http://www.cihr-irsc.gc.ca/e/7518.html, accessed July 19, 2009). Outcomes-focused knowledge translation provides an approach to knowledge translation that links patient outcomes, measurement, and feedback with research evidence and patient preferences, to encourage evidence-based practice (EBP). It involves four components:

(1) Patient outcomes measurement and feedback about outcomes achievement;
(2) Best-practice guidelines and other forms of practice evidence specific to the patient's outcome needs;
(3) Clarification of the patient's preferences for care; and
(4) Facilitation.

The outcomes-focused knowledge-translation framework was informed by the Promoting Action on Research Implementation in Health Services (PARIHS) model. Figure 4.1 illustrates the framework.

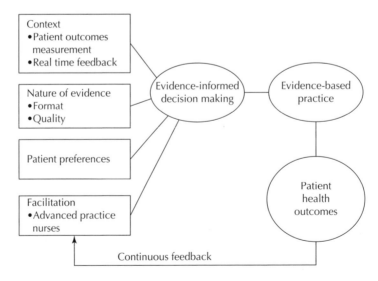

**Figure 4.1** Outcomes-focused knowledge-translation framework.
*Source*: Doran and Sidani (2007). Reprinted with the permission from Blackwell Publishing.

## Purpose of the framework

A conceptual framework is described as a set of broad ideas and principles taken from relevant fields of enquiry and used to guide research or practice. It is a set of coherent ideas or concepts organized in a manner that makes them easy to communicate to others. The outcomes-focused knowledge-translation framework was developed to guide knowledge-translation activities by encouraging the uptake of evidence through patient outcomes measurement and feedback and through reflective practice. Its primary target audience is the individual clinician. The individual clinician is a linchpin in the knowledge-translation process because it is the individual clinician who is the ultimate arbiter of decisions related to the care and treatment of patients (Brehaut et al. 2007). With new knowledge in the health sciences being advanced so rapidly, clinical practice has become the most efficient context for learning about new innovations in patient care (Handfield-Jones et al. 2002). We note that a most compelling rationale for EBP is that it offers an approach to foster learning that goes beyond ad hoc needs to true lifelong learning (Spring 2007). We also know that the individual clinician does not practice in isolation but is influenced by the action of others and by the norms, resources, and facilities of the practice environment (Rycroft-Malone et al. 2002). The context of care is most important to the translation of new knowledge. To explore how outcomes should stimulate that learning translation at the clinical level it is helpful to examine in more detail the outcomes-focused knowledge-translation framework, its theoretical foundations, and empirical evidence.

## The focus on outcomes

In its bid to increase accountability for the delivery of health-care services, to promote quality improvement, and to measure the impact of nurses within the health-care system, the Ontario Ministry of Health and Long-Term Care (MOHLTC) instituted data collection on a core set of patient outcomes that are sensitive to the practice of nurses (Pringle & White 2002). This initiative, which is known as Health Outcomes for Better Information and Care (HOBIC), involves the collection of outcomes data by nurses at the time patients are admitted to health-care services and at discharge. HOBIC consists of a set of generic outcomes relevant for adult populations in acute care, home care, long-term care, and complex continuing care settings. The HOBIC outcomes include functional status, symptoms (pain, nausea, dypsnea, fatigue), pressure ulcers, falls, and therapeutic self-care. Staff nurses are instructed in how to collect the outcomes data using standardized tools and in how to record their assessments as part of routine documentation. This Ontario initiative is highlighting the importance of patient outcomes data and is making it much more accessible to frontline providers of care. Because the outcomes are collected as part of routine practice, nurses and other clinicians have the opportunity to receive real-time feedback about patient outcomes achievement. This opportunity for real-time feedback about how patients are responding to health-care interventions provides an ideal opportunity to link real-time outcomes feedback with knowledge-translation activities.

Patient outcomes are defined as changes in the patient's health status that can be attributed to antecedent health care (Donabedian 1980). Outcomes measurement tells us about how a patient is responding to a health-care intervention but outcomes data can also be used as a basis for planning and evaluating health-care delivery. The value of outcomes research and its relevance to EBP is illustrated in the following two studies (Bernabei et al. 1998; Zyczkowska et al. 2007). Bernabei et al. followed approximately 13,000 cancer patients discharged to home from hospital and found that approximately 4000 (~29%) reported pain on a daily basis (Bernabei et al. 1998). Twenty six percent of the patients who experienced pain on a daily basis received no analgesia at all, contrary to the World Health Organization's (WHO) best-practice guideline recommendations for cancer pain management (Zech et al. 1995). A decade later we still observed problems with effective pain management. Zyczkowska et al. followed the outcomes of 193,198 home care and complex continuing care clients and found there was a consistent decline in the percentage of patients receiving analgesia consistent with the WHO best-practice recommendations among those in the highest age groups (Zyczkowska et al. 2007). Centenarians (those 100 years of age or older) made up 0.41% ($n = 788$) of the sample. Twenty percent of the clients aged 100 years and older were receiving no analgesia agents for their pain. These studies clearly demonstrate a disconnect between the knowledge, the outcomes, and the care provided. This chapter will explore how outcomes-focused knowledge-translation can be utilized to change this picture by improving EBP.

The premise underlying outcomes-focused knowledge translation is that health-care professionals will be motivated to change their practice through access to real-time feedback about their patients' outcomes and through timely access to best-practice guidelines and other forms of evidence that inform decision making. EBP is the process of shared decision making between practitioner, patient, and others significant to them based on research evidence, the patient's experiences and preferences, clinical expertise or know-how, and other available robust sources of information (Sigma Theta Tau International 2005–2007 Research and Scholarship Advisory Committee 2008: p. 57). One mechanism by which outcomes feedback is expected to improve evidence-informed decision making and treatment outcomes involves critical reflection about what is working and what is not working in patient care. A second mechanism by which outcomes feedback is expected to improve treatment outcomes may involve improved communication between the clinician and patient (Pyne & Labbate 2008). Research by Lambert suggests that patient-focused outcomes-feedback endeavors to improve outcomes by monitoring patient progress and providing this information to clinicians in order to guide ongoing treatment (Lambert et al. 2005).

## Practice reflection based on outcomes

If a patient's outcomes are not responding in the desired direction or at the expected rate of change, the outcomes feedback should encourage clinicians to reflect on their practice. With regard to such reflection, a central finding from cognitive psychology is that human reasoning can be characterized as involving two parallel forms of processing. The first form, a fast, intuitive, relatively automatic form of reasoning, can stem either from instinctual cognitive processes or from highly practiced, over-learned behavior (Brehaut et al. 2007). The second form is a slower, rational, deliberative form of reasoning. Brehaut et al. (2007) noted that knowledge structures that allow for fast, intuitive reasoning are a central component in the development of medical expertise. For novices, every decision must involve deliberative consideration of relevant signs and symptoms, while for experts many decisions can be made effortlessly (Brehaut et al. 2007). However, they further note that for all its advantages, intuitive reasoning is also subject to a well-known range of biases and contextual errors. The goal of outcomes-focused knowledge translation is to stimulate rational deliberative reasoning about the patient's response to health-care intervention and about the most appropriate patient-care interventions. Those interventions are ones that are based on the best available evidence and on patient preferences. Therefore, the aim of outcomes-focused knowledge translation is to shift practice away from unproven interventions toward EBPs.

Lockyer et al. (2004) suggested that reflection is the "engine" that shifts surface learning to deep learning and transforms knowing in action into knowledge in action. They noted that reflection changes current knowledge, experiences, and feelings into new knowledge. Practice reflection enables the clinician to gain an understanding of what is effective in a particular patient context. Evidence in combination with reflection helps the clinician to attain an understanding of the change in practice that is required.

## Outcomes feedback

The literature on cognitive psychology clearly indicates that improving performance in any complex task is dependent on feedback, in particular, feedback that is immediate and specific (Brehaut et al. 2007; Jamtvedt et al. 2003). Audit and feedback approaches involve measuring provider performance over many patients and then providing generalized feedback about how that performance stands within a distribution of other provider colleagues (Foy & Eccles 2009). This ordinarily occurs well after individual patient-care decisions have been made. However, effective performance improvement requires more immediate and specific feedback (Brehaut et al. 2007; Kluger & DeNisi 1996). Outcomes feedback provides health professionals with specific information related to the results of their work, information that is essential for improving performance (Kluger & DeNisi 1996). Care provided in the absence of knowledge of its impact, even if based on the best available evidence, can be misdirected. Furthermore, practice guidelines established for specific diagnostic groups still need to be tailored to the needs of the individual patient and adapted based on the patient's response to treatment as evidenced by the patient's outcome status (DiCenso 1999).

The effects of Feedback Intervention (FI) on performance are well documented (Axt-Adams et al. 1993; Gill et al. 1999; Heffner 2001;

Thompson O'Brien et al. 2002); however, the evidence demonstrates considerable variation in impact (Doran & Sidani 2007; Kiefe et al. 2001). Kiefe et al. (2001) have shown that providing feedback in comparison to results achieved by the best performing providers can be more effective than providing feedback comparing individuals to average results. Doran and Sidani (2007) found that FIs have primarily targeted feedback about the *processes* of care/health-care intervention. *Outcomes* feedback is identified as an important element in performance improvement that is often used in chronic disease management to provide clinicians with information about treatment outcomes (Pyne & Labbate 2008; Von Korff et al. 1997). In another care context, Slade et al. (2006) found that mental health standardized outcomes assessment, consisting of quality of life, mental health problem severity, and therapeutic alliance, along with feedback to clinicians and patients every 3 months was associated with fewer psychiatric admissions. A meta-analysis of clinical trials by Lambert and colleagues (2005), utilizing 2,500 cases, found significant improvement in psychotherapy treatment outcomes following outcomes-feedback interventions. The outcomes feedback not only reduced patient deterioration but also led to improvement in clinically meaningful outcomes (Lambert et al. 2005). Lambert et al. (2005) concluded that therapists became more attentive to a patient when they received feedback that the patient was not progressing as expected. Pyne and Labbate (2008) designed a study to determine which outcome domains were preferred by patients with schizophrenia to be included in a real-time FI. Overall, physical health problems were the most preferred outcome domain, followed by medication side effects, and satisfaction with mental health treatment. The long-term goal of Pyne and Labatte's research is to include the patient perspective in the design of real-time outcomes FI (Pyne & Labbate 2008). Through each of these studies the patient's perspective is confirmed as an important component of evidence-informed decision making.

The objective in outcomes-focused knowledge translation is to provide the feedback to clinicians at the point-of-care. Point-of-care in this context is where clinicians and patients interact and could include the bedside, an ambulatory clinic, the home, or even an electronic communication. A computerized handheld "information gathering and dissemination system" (e-Volution in Outcomes-Focused Knowledge Translation[TM]) was developed that enables nurses, simultaneously to: (a) assess and record patient outcomes information through a wireless network using personal digital assistants (PDAs) or mobile tablet personal computers (PCs); (b) present information in summary format for case-based reasoning; (c) experience real-time feedback of patient outcomes information; and (d) reference practice information, such as best-practice guidelines, at the point-of-care (Doran & Dipietro 2008; Doran et al. 2007a). In this system, feedback is provided in two formats: (i) clinicians receive feedback about change in the patient's outcomes in graphical format and (ii) clinicians have the ability to benchmark their patient's outcomes relative to similar patients. The similarity is based on medical diagnosis, co-morbidities, age, and gender. This feedback serves as a decision aid, prompting the nurse to re-evaluate the plan of care if the patient's outcomes are not improving or not changing at either the expected rate or in the expected direction. The system was evaluated in a study that engaged six settings: three hospitals and three home-care agencies. Acute care nurses in the study who used PDAs to assess patient outcomes, receive real-time feedback, and access best-practice guidelines reported that communication improved significantly. They also found that, with respect to feedback, they were more likely to receive information in a timely manner when their patient's condition changed (Doran et al. 2007b).

## Patient preferences for care

Evidence-based medicine is "the conscientious, explicit, and judicious use of current, best evidence in making decisions about the care of individual patients" (Sackett et al. 1997: p. 2). In nursing, evidence base has come to mean more than just the use of research in practice (Ciliska et al. 2001). Engaging the patient in the evidence gathering is recognized as a significant component of EBP (Coyler & Kamath 1999; Sidani et al. 2006). Coyler and Kamath (1999) proposed an approach to care that integrates the evidence base with a patient-centered focus. That integrated approach consists of identifying effective interventions, presenting the pros and cons of different treatment options to the patient, and incorporating the patient's preference in the treatment recommendation. Sidani et al. (2006) describe another patient-centered evidence-based approach to care involving three steps: identifying alternative treatment options that are found effective and relevant, on the basis of the best available evidence; consulting with patients to elicit their preference for alternative treatment options; and accounting for patients' preference in providing treatment. Treatment preference reflects the person's expression of values and attitude toward alternative interventions. In Spring's research (Spring 2007) "preferences are the lynchpin in the movement towards shared health decision-making" (p. 614). Shared decision making is defined as "a decision making process jointly shared by patients and their health care providers" (Legare et al. 2008: p. 526). A systematic review of the barriers and facilitators related to shared decision making found that the three most frequent barriers were time pressure, lack of applicability due to patient characteristics, and lack of applicability due to the clinical situation (Legare et al. 2008). The three most often identified facilitators were: (1) motivation of health professionals, (2) the perception that shared decision making will lead to a positive impact on patient outcomes, and (3) the perception that shared decision making will lead to a positive impact on the clinical process (Legare et al. 2008).

In outcomes-focused knowledge translation, clinicians engage patients systematically in treatment decision making by eliciting their preferences for care, clarifying their values, and incorporating the evidence into clinical decision making about health-care intervention. Of interest in this regard, an electronic clinical decision support system has been developed that provides clinicians with timely access to clinical evidence and feedback data about patient outcomes at the point-of-care. The system is designed to address many of the barriers to shared decision making identified by Legare et al. (2008). For example, timely access to evidence at the point-of-care addresses some of the time barriers clinicians experience because the evidence is available at the time of clinician–patient discussion. The outcomes-feedback data are important to enabling clinicians to see the positive impact of shared decision making on patient outcomes. Clinical expertise is needed to integrate the evidence from research and from patient preferences and values, and to determine the intervention/treatment that is most appropriate for the patient (Doran & Dipietro 2008; Doran et al. 2009). Patient involvement in care or treatment-related decision making has been associated with increased sense of control, increased satisfaction with care, and improved functional and clinical outcomes (McCormack et al. 1999; Street & Voigt 1997). In a study of the extent to which patients and care providers desire mutual decision making, BeLue et al. (2004) found that patient involvement in decision making is largely dependent upon the provider. "Patients look to providers to assist them in decision making and expect providers to tell them not only the full scope of treatment options but also how they can engage in clinical decision making" (Mazurek Melnyk & Fineout-Overbolt 2006: p. 125). The development of tools to measure patient preferences is a burgeoning area in medical research (Spring 2007) and should be incorporated into electronic decision support tools for use at the point-of-care.

## Facilitation to support change

Facilitation is the technique by which one person helps others to understand what they have to change and how they change it to achieve the desired outcome (Kitson et al. 1998). The facilitator role is an important component of the PARIHS model (Kitson et al. 1998; Rycroft-Malone et al. 2002). Harvey et al. (2002) noted the kinds of strategies thought to be effective in facilitating EBP. These include change management techniques such as academic detailing, educational outreach visits, audit and feedback (described earlier), social influence, and marketing approaches. They further observed that the most effective implementation strategies are those that adopt a multifaceted approach (Harvey et al. 2002). In a study of information behavior in the context of improving patient safety, McIntosh-Murray and Choo (2005) found advanced practice nurses performed an important role as "information/ change agent" for inpatient nursing teams. The functions of the information/change agent included: (a) acting as a *boundary spanner* between the front-line staff nurses' patient level of focus and the system-process level and between staff nurses and resources outside the unit; (b) acting as an *information seeker* for frontline staff nurses and seeking appropriate information; and (c) acting as a *change champion* with "just-in-time" education, change initiatives, and ongoing coaching. In the Advancing Research and Clinical Practice through close Collaboration (ARCC) model the facilitator is referred to as an EBP mentor (Mazurek Melnyk & Fineout-Overbolt 2006). Mazurek Melnyk and Fineout-Overbolt (2006) describe the elements of the EBP mentor role as providing knowledge and skills about research to others, assisting others to hone their skills in assessing patient preferences, and incorporating patient preferences into clinical decision making.

In outcomes-focused knowledge translation, facilitation involves each of the characteristics described earlier. It also draws on techniques and approaches from quality-improvement literature and from learning theory. From that literature we know that the facilitator needs to assist staff in interpreting significant trends in outcome achievement by utilizing the theory of statistical process control (Berwick 1991; Deming 1986). Facilitation should include the broad participation of clinicians, managers, and other staff involved in delivering care, in measurement and statistical analysis, in problem solving through inductive reasoning, and in progress through small-scale implementation and evaluation (Herman et al. 2006). Facilitation must engage all participants in the cognitive aspects of care. "Cognitive learning often involves seeing a problem from a new perspective or viewpoint. Change requires cognitive re-organization and perhaps even the abandonment of previously learned principles or approaches" (Handfield-Jones et al. 2002: p. 951).

Self-determination theory (SDT) (Ryan & Deci 2000) is a well-established and validated theory of adult motivation that pertains to the role of facilitation in achieving change. It has direct implications for adult learning through the insights it provides into how motivation relates to three of the basic psychological needs of individuals: autonomy, competence, and relatedness. It posits that humans search out growth opportunities and naturally seek to engage in meaningful activities, to enhance capabilities, and to encounter social connectedness in groups. SDT explicitly addresses the social environment of the individual striving to realize the goals of growth, improvement, and self-actualization. The social environment must support and nourish human growth-oriented endeavors. The facilitator role is an important component of the social environment because facilitators need to create a favorable learning environment where clinicians experience autonomy, competence, and relatedness in order to achieve practice change.

## Related theoretical models

## Model A. Promoting Action on Research Implementation in Health Services

Outcomes–focused knowledge translation is based in cognitive learning theory (Kluger & DeNisi 1996; Ryan & Deci 2000) and was conceptualized as an approach to operationalize the concepts from the PARIHS model (Kitson et al. 1998; Rycroft-Malone et al. 2002) at the point-of-care. The PARIHS model provides a framework for guiding the continuous improvement of nursing practice through EBP (Kitson et al. 1998; Rycroft-Malone et al. 2002). Kitson et al. (1998) suggest that successful implementation of evidence into practice is a function of the relationship between (a) the nature of the evidence, (b) the context in which practice change will occur, and (c) the mechanisms by which the change is facilitated. They describe the *nature* of evidence in three formats: research information, clinical experience, and patient choice. Successful implementation into practice is most likely when the research evidence is of high quality, where there is high professional consensus concerning the evidence, and where there is a process for systematic feedback and input from patients into health-care decision making. The *context* is the environment or setting in which the proposed change will be implemented. It consists of three elements: the prevailing culture, the leadership roles assigned, and measurement, that is the organization's approach to monitoring its systems and services. *Facilitation*, as previously indicated, is the technique by which one person helps others to understand what they have to change and how they change it to achieve the desired outcome (Kitson et al. 1998).

Practice development, as conceptualized by Kitson and colleagues, involves the continuous improvement of patient care through EBP (Kitson 2002; McCormack et al. 1999). The PARIHS model is helpful in identifying the important elements within the practice setting that need to be in place in order to foster EBP change. It identifies performance measurement as an important component of the context for change. However, previous descriptions of the model do not specifi-cally identify which indicators are appropriate for evaluating nursing systems and services or how to use performance measurement and feedback to design and evaluate practice change. Outcomes-focused knowledge translation provides a framework to operationalize the performance measurement and feedback component of the PARIHS model. As such, it is complimentary to the PARIHS model. It should be applied in conjunction with the other knowledge-translation strategies identified within the PARIHS model. Indeed, evidence suggests that without such a multifaceted set of interventions and strategies, knowledge translation will be less successful (Graham et al. 2006).

In outcomes-focused knowledge translation patient outcomes feedback and research evidence are linked through an electronic decision support system that is designed to support evidence-informed decision making at the point-of-care. A theory-driven approach has been used to develop the decision-support system. Building on the suggestions in the PARIHS model, research findings are provided in the form of best-practice guidelines and are presented to clinicians in a "push" fashion, automatically, in response to their outcomes assessment data. Previous research suggests that it may be more effective to provide clinicians with research evidence in a "push" fashion that is automatically delivered in the form of alerts and reminders, than in a "pull" fashion, that relies on clinicians to search out the information (Bates et al. 2003). Consistent with the recommendations in the PARIHS model, a hyperlink is provided within the knowledge-translation system that enables clinicians to read about the quality of the evidence and its source. The inclusion of a discussion of the quality of the evidence and its source is thought to function as a social-persuasion mechanism, anticipating that clinicians are more likely to adopt evidence in practice when they believe the evidence comes from a credible source and is of high quality.

## Model B. Knowledge-to-Action

Outcomes-focused knowledge translation can also fit within a broader framework for knowledge-to-action (KTA) developed by Graham et al. (2006). KTA is a process for practice change that consists of two concepts: knowledge creation and action (see Figure 4.2). Within KTA, knowledge is seen to be primarily empirically derived (i.e., research based) but also encompasses other forms of knowing such as experiential knowledge. The knowledge concept, represented by the funnel in Figure 4.2, represents knowledge creation and consists of the major types of knowledge or research, namely, primary research, knowledge synthesis (e.g., meta-analysis), and knowledge tools and products (e.g., best-practice guidelines, decision-support tools) (Graham et al. 2006). As knowledge moves through the funnel it becomes more distilled and refined. Knowledge *inquiry* represents the multitude of primary studies or information of variable quality. This is referred to as first-generation knowledge that is in its natural state. Knowledge *synthesis*, or second-generation knowledge, represents the aggregation of existing knowledge. At this stage the knowledge often takes the form of systematic reviews. Knowledge *tools* or products are third-generation knowledge and most often take the form of practice guidelines, decision aids, and rules.

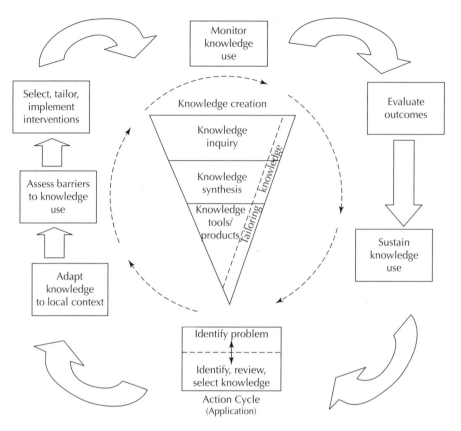

**Figure 4.2** Knowledge-to-action framework.
Reprinted, with permission, from Graham, I. D., Logan, J., Harrison, M. B., Straus, S. E., Tetroe, J., CaswellL, W. & Robinson, N. (2006) 'Lost in knowledge translation: time for a map'. *The Journal of Continuing Education in the Health Professions*, **26**, 13–24.

Outcomes-focused knowledge translation most often utilizes third-generation knowledge, that is, practice guidelines embedded in decision-support tools that deliver research evidence in response to patient outcomes data. It incorporates two major sources of knowledge for evidence-informed decision making: (i) patient outcomes data and (ii) research evidence. Recently Doran has also explored the value of providing clinicians with access to first-generation knowledge via point-of-care technologies such as PDAs (Doran 2009). For example, McMaster PLUS and Nursing PLUS (McMaster University Health Information Research Unit 2008) deliver e-mail alerts to clinicians about new research studies relevant to their clinical interest. The research studies delivered have been pre-graded for validity and clinical relevance. Clinicians are able to use PDAs, desktop computers, or laptop computers to access the e-mail alerts and to read the research abstracts from McMaster/Nursing PLUS. The nurses engaged in Doran's study found this form of access to research evidence to be timely and relevant to their practice (Doran 2009).

In the KTA framework, the term *action* is used rather than *practice* because it is seen to be more generic and encompasses the use of or application of knowledge by practitioners, policy makers, patients, and the public. Therefore the action part of the KTA process results in implementation or application of new knowledge. Graham et al. (2006) suggest the "action" phase typically begins with the identi-fication of a problem that needs addressing. In outcomes-focused knowledge translation, the problem would be a gap between the desired outcome and an observed outcome, as determined by out-comes feedback. The next phase in the action process involves the identification, review, and selection of knowledge or research relevant to the problem. As noted above, this could involve first-generation, second-generation, or third-generation knowledge. In the context of outcomes-focused knowledge translation, the knowledge component typically involves third-generation knowledge; however, other forms of knowledge have also been incorporated into decision-support tools at the point-of-care. This phase would also involve knowledge of patient preferences. In the KTA framework, Graham et al. (2006) suggest that, in the next phase, decision makers would adapt the knowledge to the local context, assess barriers to using the knowledge, select or tailor the implementation of interventions, monitor knowledge use, evaluate outcomes, and sustain ongoing knowledge use. In out-comes-focused knowledge translation these steps in the process most closely align with incorporating patient preferences into shared deci-sion making (i.e., adapting the knowledge and assessing barriers), resulting in evidence-informed decision making (i.e., deciding to act on the evidence) and EBP (i.e., tailoring the implementation of inter-ventions based on the relevant knowledge). The interactive feedback loop in Figure 4.1 represents the final process whereby outcomes are re-assessed (i.e., evaluating the outcomes of putting the knowledge to use) to determine whether the intervention is successful. In KTA, as each action phase can be influenced by the phases that precede it, there may also be feedback between the phases; thus, change may occur at each phase in the process of KTA (Graham et al. 2006).

## Conclusion

In conclusion, outcomes-focused knowledge translation was devel-oped as a model to guide knowledge translation at the point-of-care.

It involves four components: (1) patient outcomes measurement and feedback about outcomes achievement; (2) best-practice guidelines and other forms of evidence specific to the patient's outcome needs; (3) clarification of the patient's preferences for care; and (4) facilitation. The outcomes-focused knowledge-translation framework was informed by the PARIHS model. It is also complementary to the KTA framework proposed by Graham et al. (2006). It has been used to guide research related to knowledge translation at the point-of-care in acute hospital settings, home-care settings, and mental health inpatient settings (Doran 2009; Doran & Dipietro 2008; Doran et al. 2007a, 2009). Results from recent research indicate that it is feasible to provide patient outcomes feedback to clinicians at the point-of-care via electronic information terminals and thus to link outcomes feedback with research evidence to support evidence-informed decision making. However, effective change in the practice of care requires attending to the external context and to engaging facilitators who can model, lead, and reinforce practice change. Therefore, outcomes-focused knowledge translation should be introduced in conjunction with other proven knowledge-translation strategies intentionally designed to create a favorable environment for encouraging practice change.

# References

Axt-Adams, P., Van Der Wouden, J., & Van Der Does, E. (1993). Influence behaviour of physicians ordering laboratory tests: A literature study. *Medical Care*, 31, 784–794.

Bates, D.W., Kuperman, G.J., Wang, S. et al. (2003). Ten commandments for effective clinical decision support: Making the practice of evidence-based medicine a reality. *Journal of the American Medical Informatics Association*, 10, 523–530.

Belue, R., Butler, J., & Kuder, J. (2004). Implications of patient and physician decision making: An illustration in treatment options for coronary artery disease. *Journal of Ambulatory Care Management*, 27, 305–313.

Bernabei, R., Gambassi, G., Lapane, F. et al. (1998). Management of pain in elderly patients with cancer. *JAMA: the Journal of the American Medical Association*, 279, 1877–1882.

Berwick, D.M. (1991). Controlling variation in health care: A consultation from Walter Shewhart. *Medical Care*, 29, 1212–1225.

Brehaut, J.C., Hamm, R., Majumdar, S., Papa, F., & Lott, A. (2007). Cognitive and social issues in emergency medicine knowledge translation: A research agenda. *Academic Emergency Medicine*, 14, 984–990.

Ciliska, D.K., Pinelli, J., Dicenso, A., & Cullum, N. (2001). Resources to enhance evidence-based nursing practice. *AACN Clinical Issues*, 12, 520–528.

Coyler, H. & Kamath, P. (1999). Evidence based practice: A philosophical and political analysis: Some matters for consideration by professional practitioners. *Journal of Advanced Nursing*, 29, 188–193.

Deming, W.E. (1986). *Out of the Crisis*. Cambridge, MA: Massachusetts Institute of Technology.

Dicenso, A. (1999). Evidenced-based medicine, evidenced-based nursing. *Expert Nurse*, 15, 92–97.

Donabedian, A. (1980). *The Definition of Quality and Approaches to its Assessment*. Ann Arbor, MI: Health Administration Press.

Doran, D.M. (2009). The emerging role of PDAs in information use and clinical decision making. *Evidence Based Nursing*, 12, 35–38.

Doran, D.M. & Dipietro, T. (2008). Knowledge translation in nursing through decision support at the point of care. In: A. Kushniruk & E. Borycki (eds) *The Human and Social Side of Health Information Systems*. Hurshy, NY: Medical Information Science Reference.

Doran, D.M., Haynes, R.B., Straus, S. et al. (2009). Evaluation of mobile information technology to improve nurses' access to and use of research evidence. Interim report submitted to the Ministry of Health and Long-Term Care. Toronto, ON: University of Toronto.

Doran, D.M., Mylopoulos, J., Kushniruk, A. et al. (2007a). Evidence in the palm of your hand: development of an outcome-focused knowledge translation intervention. *Worldviews on Evidence-Based Nursing*, 4, 1–9.

Doran, D.M., Mylopoulos, J., Kushniruk, A. et al. (2007b). Outcomes in the palm of your hand: Improving the quality and continuity of patient care. Final Report Ontario Centres of Excellence, Ministry of Health and Long-Term Care, Canadian Institutes of Health Research. Toronto.

Doran, D.M. & Sidani, S. (2007). Outcomes focused knowledge translation: A framework for knowledge translation and patient outcomes improvement. *Worldviews on Evidence-Based Nursing*, 4, 3–13.

Foy, R. & Eccles, M. (2009). Audit and feedback interventions. In: I. Graham & J. Tetroe (eds) *Knowledge Translation in Health Care: Moving from Evidence to Practice*. Oxford: Wiley-Blackwell.

Gill, P., Makela, M., Vermeulen, K. et al. (1999). Changing doctor prescribing behaviour. *Pharmacy World & Science*, 21, 158–167.

Graham, I.D., Logan, J., Harrison, M.B. et al. (2006). Lost in knowledge translation: Time for a map. *The Journal of Continuing Education in the Health Professions*, 26, 13–24.

Handfield-Jones, R.S., Mann, K.V., Challis, M.E. et al. (2002) Linking assessment to learning: A new route to quality assurance in medical practice. *Medical Education*, 36, 949–958.

Harvey, G., Loftus-Hills, A., Rycroft-Malone, J. et al. (2002) Getting evidence into practice: The role and function of facilitation. *Journal of Advanced Nursing*, 37, 577–588.

Heffner, J.E. (2001). Altering physician behavior to improve clinical performance. *Topics in Health Information Management*, 22, 1–9.

Herman, R.C., Chan, J.A., Zazzali, J.L., & Lerner, D. (2006). Aligning measurement-based quality improvement with implementation of evidence-based practices. *Administration and Policy in Mental Health*, 33, 636–645.

Jamtvedt, G., Young, J., Kristoffersen, D., O'Brien, M., & Oxman, A. (2003). Audit and feedback: Effects on professional practice and health care outcomes (review). *The Cochrane Database of Systematic Reviews*, 3.

Kiefe, C.I., Allison, J.J., Williams, O.D., Person, S.D., Weaver, M.T., & Weissman, N.W. (2001). Improving quality improvement using achievable benchmarks for physician feedback. A randomized controlled trial. *JAMA: the Journal of the American Medical Association*, 285, 2871.

Kitson, A. (2002). Recognising relationships: Reflections on evidence-based practice. *Nursing Inquiry*, 9, 179–186.

Kitson, A., Harvey, G., & Mccormack, B. (1998). Approaches to implementing research in practice. *Quality in Health Care*, 7, 149–159.

Kluger, A.N. & Denisi, A. (1996). The effects of feedback interventions on performance: A historical review, a meta-analysis, and a preliminary feedback intervention theory. *Psychological Bulletin*, 119, 254–284.

Lambert, M.J., Harmon, C., Slade, K., Whipple, J.L., & Hawkins, E.J. (2005). Providing feedback to psychotherapists on their patients' progress: Clinical results and practice suggestions. *Journal of Clinical Psychology*, 61, 165–174.

Legare, F., Ratte, S., Gravel, K. & Graham, I.D. (2008). Barriers and facilitators to implementing shared decision-making in clinical practice: Update of a systematic review of health professionals' perceptions. *Patient Education and Counseling*, 73, 526–535.

Lockyer, J., Gondocz, S.T., & Thivierge, R.L. (2004). Knowledge translation: The role and place of practice reflection. *The Journal of Continuing Education in the Health Professions*, 24(1), 50–56.

MacIntosh-Murray, A. & Choo, C.W. (2005). Informational behavior in the context of improving patient safety. *Journal of the American Society for Information Science and Technology*, 56(12), 1332–1345.

Mazurek Melnyk, B. & Fineout-Overbolt, E. (2006). Consumer preferences and values as an integral key to evidence-based practice. *Nursing Administration Quarterly*, 30, 123–127.

Mccormack, B., Manley, K., Kitson, A., Titchen, A., & Harvey, G. (1999). Towards practice development—a vision in reality or a reality without vision? *Journal of Nursing Management*, 7, 255–264.

McMaster University Health Information Research Unit (2008). Nursing + —Best evidence for nursing care. McMaster University, Hamilton, ON Canada, Available online: http://plus.mcmaster.ca/np/Default.aspx.

Pringle, D.M. & White, P. (2002). Happenings. Nursing matters: The Nursing and Health Outcomes Project of the Ontario Ministry of Health and Long-Term Care. *Canadian Journal of Nursing Research*, 33, 115–121.

Pyne, J.M. & Labbate, C. (2008). Ranking of outcome domains for use in real-time outcomes feedback laboratory by patients with schizophrenia. *The Journal of Nervous and Mental Disease*, 196, 336–339.

Ryan, R.M. & Deci, E.L. (2000). Self-determination theory and the facilitation of intrinsic motivation, social development, and well-being. *American Psychologist*, 55, 68–78.

Rycroft-Malone, J., Kitson, A., Harvey, G. et al. (2002). Ingredients for change: Revisiting a conceptual framework. *Quality and Safety in Health Care*, 11, 174–180.

Sackett, D.L., Richardson, W.S., Rosenberg, W.M., & Haynes, R.B. (1997). *Evidence-Based Medicine: How to Practice Teach EBM*, New York: Churchill Livingstone.

Sidani, S., Epstein, D., & Miranda, J. (2006). Eliciting patient treatment preferences: A strategy to integrate evidence-based and patient centered care. *Worldviews on Evidence-Based Nursing*, 3, 1–8.

Sigma Theta Tau International 2005–2007 Research and Scholarship Advisory Committee (2008). Sigma theta tau international position statement on evidence-based practice February 2007 summary. *Worldviews on Evidence-Based Nursing*, 5, 57–59.

Slade, M., Mccrone, P., Kuipers, E. et al. (2006). Use of standardised outcome measures in adult mental health services. *British Journal of Psychiatry*, 189, 330–336.

Spring, B. (2007). Evidence-based practice in clinical psychology: What it is, why it matters; what you need to know. *Journal of Clinical Psychology*, 63, 611–631.

Street, R.L. & Voigt, B. (1997). Patient participation in deciding breast cancer treatment and subsequent quality of life. *Medical Decision Making*, 17, 298–306.

Thompson O'Brien, M., Oxman, A., Davis, D., Haynes, R., Freemantle, N., & Harvey, E. (2002). Audit and feedback versus alternative strategies: Effects on professional practice and health care outcomes. *The Cochrane Library*, 1–18.

Von Korff, M., Gruman, J., Schaefer, J., Curry, S.J., & Wagner, E.H. (1997). Collaborative management of chronic disease. *Annuals of Internal Medicine*, 127, 1097–1102.

Zech, D.F.J., Grond, S., Lynch, J., Hertel, D., & Lehmann, K. (1995). Validation of World Health Organization guidelines for cancer pain relief: A 10-year prospective study. *Pain*, 63, 65–76.

Zyczkowska, J., Szczerbinska, K., Jantzi, M.R., & Hirdes, J.P. (2007). Pain among the oldest old in community and institutional settings. *Pain*, 129, 167–176.

# Chapter 5

# Outcomes of evidence-based practice: practice to policy perspectives

## Examples from the field of chronic wounds

*Margaret B. Harrison*

---

**Key learning points**

- Implementation of evidence-based practice is typically complex, time consuming, and resource intensive and the importance of measuring outcomes is twofold: to evaluate the effectiveness of the change in practice and plan for its sustainability.
- Outcome concepts can usually be measured in various ways—the choice is a balance between scientific rigor and feasibility.
- Implementation teams need to take into account multiple perspectives with outcome selection considering individual/family, provider, and system-level measures.

---

## Introduction

Implementation of evidence-based practice (EBP) is often complex, time consuming, and resource intensive. The importance of measuring outcomes is vital not only to evaluate the effectiveness of the change in practice, but also to invest in its sustainability. To accomplish this, implementation teams should consider evaluation and outcome selection from multiple perspectives. This chapter describes the types of outcome measures that can be used to evaluate implementation of EBP. Approaches to measurement, key outcome concepts, and selection of measurement methods will be presented, as well as the strengths and limitations of different approaches. The chapter describes a program of research focused on evidence-based implementation with chronic wound practices (pressure ulcers and leg ulcers) to illustrate the different purposes of these outcome measures, their effects on knowledge use by providers, and the impact on patients, providers, and the health system.

## Background

During the mid-1990s the availability of quality practice guidelines provided a crucial impetus for the "best practice" movement. Settings and providers now had access to evidence in a useable form that could potentially be integrated into practice-based decision making to improve outcomes. The long-held notion of "that's the way it has always been done" could and would be challenged. However, the reality of *basing practice on best available evidence* was far more difficult than any of us imagined.

Many nursing settings first actively experienced implementation of EBP to improve both the prevention and management of pressure ulcers. Pressure ulcers present a ubiquitous problem that cross sectors of care and patient populations and are, for the most part, deemed a nursing concern. Chronic leg ulcers provided another opportunity for implementation. Again, nurses deliver the majority of leg ulcer care to a population largely based in the community. With more than a dozen years beyond these early implementation initiatives in nursing, it has become increasingly clear how vital the evaluation, meticulous tailoring, and selection of outcomes in implementing EBP is to the whole process. The instrumental role that outcome measures can play will be illustrated using chronic wound cases as exemplars.

Members of our research team spanned a large Ontario health region in central Canada. The team first came together in the mid-1990s to implement practice guidelines for pressure ulcer prevention and management. Originally the effort was concentrated in acute care in one large teaching hospital but soon led to a diverse regional collaboration in different settings across the continuum of care. Around the same time, we undertook a second major initiative related to best practice with community-based leg ulcer care. With both examples a substantive research and quality component accompanied the guideline implementations. Much was learned about translating knowledge to practice, exposing the gap between having quality guidelines and actual implementation and the challenges with outcome measurement. Using these chronic wound cases I will highlight what worked in our efforts and what did not, and postulate the reasons why. The journey was rarely straightforward.

## Building the case for change for EBP

### Prevalence/incidence rates as outcome, the process as a monitoring mechanism

In both examples of pressure and leg ulcer EBP implementation, work began by determining the extent of the problem. The key questions facing us were, "How widespread were the problems/issues, and what were the profiles of the at-risk population"? Multiple sectors in our Eastern Ontario health-care region (population ~1 million) were engaged in a concerted effort to address issues related to pressure ulcer occurrence. Initial research to assess the extent of the problem and evaluate a risk assessment tool in a hospital setting provided the methodological foundation and practical tools to collect prevalence estimates (Fisher et al. 1996; Harrison et al. 1996). Because little occurrence information was available in administrative databases to understand the extent and severity of the problem, our group decided its first step must be the collection of primary data over time. This long-range study was, in turn, the basis of ongoing monitoring activity and the ongoing surveillance that resulted in yearly prevalence studies across the institution. "Prevalence" included a full head-to-toe skin assessment and risk profile using a recommended risk tool. The monitoring activity diffused into other settings and over time, and became a reliable, valid, and clinically feasible monitoring process. To participate in the prevalence data collection, surveyors were trained in comprehensive skin assessment and use of the risk tool. The education workshop included both theoretical and practical "hands-on" components in staging pressure ulcers. And, to evaluate our ability to collect this data, a validation team of two experienced surveyors reassessed a 10% reference sample of the prevalence population. The evaluation showed a strong relationship between the initial and reference sample assessments (Harrison et al. 1996).

The prevalence data collection provided the structure for a comprehensive local dataset from which to derive benchmarks and continue evaluating changes to care. For instance, the prevalence and incidence hospital data were analyzed and reported across the health-care setting, at the levels of hospital, program, and unit. Specific units with high chronic wound occurrences conducted more in-depth studies of their own patients and contextual factors with assistance from the nursing quality portfolio (Mackey et al. 2005). Over time the portfolio was used in different ways to drive the quality and continuing effort with EBP (Harrison 2008; Harrison et al. 1998). Quality monitoring processes emerged from the prevalence and incidence methodologies, providing the foundation from which care changes for improved pressure ulcer outcomes could be advocated. Incremental improvement could be tracked by specific ulcer stage indicating that although the overall prevalence may not have decreased, the severity of the problem had improved at a population level.

Like pressure ulcers, leg ulcers fall primarily under nursing purview. Again, little data was available from agency administrative databases. To gain an accurate picture of precisely how many individuals in the catchment area suffered from leg ulcers, and how many were potentially coming into care, it was again necessary to conduct prevalence, incidence, and profiling studies before implementation of recommendations from international guidelines could begin. Information was lacking about their numbers or their circumstances (age, mobility, progress of care). Because we were unable to find any Canadian epidemiology studies of this condition, we conducted a substantive review of international studies that documented rates and methodologies used to measure the problem (Graham et al. 2003a). To create a benchmark and produce this data for local decision makers and planners, we undertook a 1-month prospective study that included a full clinical assessment comprising an ankle-brachial pressure index, clinical history, socio-demographic and circumstance-of-living information. The attending nurse collected the information on a planned visit. This provided a composite of data of baseline statistics and benchmarks from which to assess future care and community management of this population (Graham et al. 2003a,b).

## Understanding the environment and current care

### Context and process of care, setting up process outcomes

Once the intended population to receive the evidence-informed care and services has been identified, the next task is typically to understand the context and provider practices. Environmental scans, provider knowledge, attitudes, practice (KAP) surveys, and process audits can all be useful approaches. Outcomes from these approaches include: the readiness of the environment and providers to implement changes, and the gap between current practice and best practice that must be addressed. In the case of pressure ulcers, an internal quality audit of patient charts revealed no consistent or standardized risk assessment for pressure ulcer risk. If a pressure ulcer was diagnosed, it was largely managed following a referral to the hospital-wide consultant, an enterostomal therapist. Yet the guidelines we followed at that time, the Agency of Health Care Policy and Research (1992) guideline recommendations, clearly advocated for identification of people at risk. To accomplish this, ongoing regular assessments must be conducted by regular, ongoing caregivers, that is, by bedside staff rather than consultants, to determine risk (Agency for Healthcare Research and Quality, AHCPR, 1992).

To assist us in meeting the many challenges raised by this implementation, we were guided by a research use framework to improve our ability to overcome barriers and make fruitful use of facilitating factors (Logan et al. 1999). The framework, the Ottawa Model of Research Use, helps us focus on important provider, environment, and guideline factors. For example, one barrier that became evident was nurses' lack of knowledge and skill in using risk assessment tools. A training program was developed to assist nurses in the use of risk scales recommended in the guideline (AHCPR 1992). Guidelines provide a roadmap only. How the recommendations are enacted in a particular setting requires attention to the environmental details and articulation within a care protocol. When our audits indicated the need for a more visible outcome, a skin care task force was formed to review documentation and develop a mechanism to record assessment on the daily vital signs flow sheet within patients' charts. This had the effect of improving documentation allowing for quality audits to track the number and timing of risk assessments, the proportion of patients "at risk," how severe the risk was, and provided the potential to link this information to preventative interventions.

Quality process outcomes (instrumental knowledge use or indicators) are important to providing a barometer of how well guideline recommendations are being adhered to in a setting.

In the case of community leg ulcer care, authority and decision-making capacity is held at both the individual provider and regional levels. A KAP survey of nurses and family physicians (Graham et al. 2001, 2003b) supplied a crucial impetus for the home-care authority to appreciate the willingness of providers to adhere to a regionally driven protocol. Once a referral was received for home-care services, a locally adapted evidence protocol outlined the plan of care (Graham et al. 2000); exceptions were made only by physician order. The KAP survey also brought to light existing gaps in provider skills and knowledge. Knowledge outcomes (conceptual knowledge use) for instance directed to the areas of evidence where physicians and nurses required more support. For example, additional effort was required to improve providers' evidence-informed assessment capability. Nurses required training and equipment to carry this out. A key aspect of conducting a comprehensive clinical evaluation included performing an ankle-brachial pressure measurement index (ABPI) using handheld Dopplers. This was not standard equipment at the time for home-nursing agencies. Later these aspects (the availability of equipment, training incorporated in new staff nurse orientations) would be tracked as a process outcome in adhering to the guideline recommendations.

Another important outcome to come to light in the early stages of the leg ulcer best practice implementation project was system outcome such as resource use (Friedberg et al. 2002). This included administratively important outcomes such as nursing time, the number of visits, types and costs of supplies and equipment. In later evaluation efforts, these outcomes were influential for decision makers to make judgments about continuing with the newly organized service.

## Measuring the impact of EBP/care

## Evaluations and selecting practice and health services outcomes

Evaluations of implementation projects are an artful dance between rigor, timeliness, and feasibility. Planners and decision makers typically have a short window of opportunity to inform decisions, and evaluative data must be responsive to this reality. Often there is no time to wait for the perfect evaluation study. In the chronic wound examples presented in this chapter, implementations were evaluated from an integrated researcher, practitioner, and decision-maker perspective. For instance, the providers were largely interested in improving the wound to a point where day-to-day function was near normal. Decision makers were interested in reasonable periods of time on service and when improvement and coming off-service were feasible. From a research perspective, time-to-healing is considered a sensitive wound outcome. Thus given the chronic nature of leg ulcers, a 3-month healing rate was a reasonable compromise. Outcomes selection also needed to include system-level indicators of less interest to frontline providers. For instance, in both wound cases healing was an important clinical outcome, yet efficiencies and use of scarce resources (e.g., nursing time) were key for decision makers choosing between priorities. Needless to say, many challenges are faced at this stage of implementation both methodologically and practically.

Pressure ulcer outcomes were selected/derived from the original monitoring process using prevalence and incidence methodologies. Outcomes used in the hospital included: prevalence estimates, types and severity of risk based on 6 risk subscales (Bergstrom et al. 1987; Braden 1987) stages of ulcer from less to most severe. Prevalence estimates became a hospital-wide quality indicator. Risk profiles are used at unit level to plan intervention strategies (e.g., for moisture or mobility deficits). Outcomes indicating improvement rather than healing are also used (e.g., fewer of the severe ulcers using the National Pressure Ulcer Advisory Panel (1989) staging classification). One additional measure that has been added is the assessment of patient-reported pain with pressure ulcers (Girouard et al. 2008).

Work has continued to evaluate trends over time using the adverse event of pressure ulcer occurrence (Vandenkerkhof et al. 2005). Although helpful as a setting-wide indicator, prevalence estimates are limited in their usefulness to actual decision making in practice. Prevalence information does not shed light on when pressure ulcers are likely to occur, or the factors that contribute to their occurrence, deterioration, or improvement. To gain insight in these areas, ongoing, real-time, incidence data collection, rather than prevalence estimates, is required. Unlike prevalence performed as a one-shot cross-sectional effort, incidence data requires regular day-to-day tracking with established periodic analyses (weekly, monthly, and/or quarterly). This is particularly important for units with higher pressure ulcer occurrence. Although incidence rates have been periodically undertaken in our setting (Graham et al. 2004; Mackey et al. 2005), time and resource constraints continue to make this a challenge.

In the community leg ulcer example, outcomes were based on a combination of clinical and system-level concepts. In a 1-year pre-post study (Harrison et al. 2005), the primary healing outcome, a 3-month healing rate, was selected for comparative and feasibility reasons. The 3-month rate for leg ulcer studies was used predominantly in the international literature. Importantly it was a practical outcome for the service team to collect and use with this slow healing wound. After implementation of the evidence-based protocol, healing more than doubled going from 23% to 56% ($p = \ < 0.001$) (Harrison et al. 2005). System outcomes, including the number of nursing visits per case, declined from a median of 37 to 25 ($p = 0.041$). The median supply cost per case was reduced from $1,923 to $406 Canadian ($p = 0.005$).

In a further study, undertaken by the same team, a randomized control trial compared and evaluated clinical and cost-effectiveness of home-versus-nurse clinic delivery of evidence-based care leg ulcer care using a health systems perspective (Harrison et al. 2008). In an era of economic constraints, this was a pressing issue for regional health-care authorities and home-nursing agencies in decisions about instituting nurse-led clinics for some client groups. In this trial we found no differences in the healing outcomes at 3 months (clinic 58.3%; home 56.7%) nor with any of the secondary outcomes which included durability of healing (time before next ulcer episode), recurrence within 1 year, health-related quality of life, patient satisfaction with care (short survey), and resource use (number of visits, supply expenditures). The study revealed that organizing care to deliver evidence-based care was key to achieving positive health and system outcomes not the location or setting of care (home versus clinic). Thus, regional community care authorities can use either home or clinic care to provide leg ulcer services and expect similar results. The modality of delivery is a decision on what may be appropriate for their community and resource availability.

Self-reported outcomes among individuals who are the recipients of care have become more important in leg ulcer implementation studies. Quality of life, satisfaction with care, and pain with this condition have been explored from a research perspective and integrated as part of the quality processes. The tools used to measure these outcomes are described in detail elsewhere but suffice to say they were selected for their clinical sensibility and feasibility. Health-related quality of life and pain are both measured with short form tools. For example, Nemeth and colleagues (2003a) adapted a rigorous process for assessing pain in this community population using a two-step method, followed by studies to examining impact of this symptom in order to improve nursing management (Nemeth et al. 2003b). The pain assessment method was embedded in the documentation so that it could be quality audited and nurse adherence to evidence recommendations followed as a natural course during the plan of care.

Our most recent trial related to the evidence-based leg ulcer program of research is focused on two high-compression technologies to establish which is superior (effective and efficient) in the community setting (Harrison et al. 2003). In this trial, a health services outcome was selected as most appropriate. This trial evaluated differences in healing with use of two common compression bandaging systems where the primary outcome was a 5-week or greater difference in healing. Clinically, time-to-healing is the outcome of choice and the 5-week difference serves as a health services outcome identified as relevant by service providers. The 5-week outcome was arrived at through consultation with home-care and nursing agency authorities and based on supply expenditures and nursing time involved in delivering each of these technologies. The 5-week difference in healing rates was deemed the tipping point to influence any decision to switch from one bandaging technology to the other. Otherwise, both would be considered effective and efficient and remain available on the supply inventories.

## Limitations of different approaches

There are "pluses" and "minuses" of the various approaches to outcome assessment with an EBP implementation. One is typically trading off rigor with clinical sensibility and feasibility. One may want to conduct a full-scale resource use study but the practicality is that you have a limited amount of expenditure data in administrative databases that will be easy to capture and lend itself to modeling to impute full costs. In Table 5.1, a summary of the major

**Table 5.1** Outcomes used with evidence-based practice implementation for two chronic wound populations (pressure ulcers and leg ulcers)

| | Outcome concept | Measure | Strengths, limitations |
|---|---|---|---|
| **Individual** | Healing | Time-to-healing | Sensitive, time consuming, resource intensive, widely used, relatively easy to collect |
| | | 3-month rate | |
| | Improvement in wound | Reduction in size or stage | Sensitive when overall prevalence does not vary greatly, reliability with different providers may be challenging |
| | Durability of healing | Recurrence following last ulcer healed | Excellent information for service planning, resource intensive to follow individuals |
| | Pain | Numeric Rating Scale (NRS) | Both NRS and VAS are simple, efficient, valid, and reliable measures. If pain is present a more detailed assessment of the quality of pain is required |
| | | Visual Analogue Scale (VAS) | |
| | | McGill Pain Scale | |
| | Satisfaction with care | Short survey developed for specific EBP recommendations | Quick and simple to elicit feedback, may provide helpful planning information |
| **Provider** | Provider characteristics | KAP survey | Useful to contextualize the local protocol, may be difficult to administer if trying to reach all affected providers |
| | Satisfaction with professional practice | Short survey developed for specific EBP recommendations | Quick and simple to elicit feedback, may provide helpful planning information |
| **System** | Reduction in Problem | Prevalence Estimates | Setting/service wide surveys are resource intensive for primary data collection, audited data may not be reliable |
| | Resource Use | Expenditures per case of supplies and nursing time | Fairly simple, readily available data, may be used for more sophisticated economic analyses |
| | | # visits per episode of care | |
| | | Readmission to service | |

outcomes used in the chronic wound implementations is provided with the strengths and limitations of the outcomes. It is important to remember that for any one outcome concept there are usually several means to capture the information. The best measure may carry too high a burden of administration presenting the risk of incomplete data for decision makers. The researcher, clinician, and decision-maker and service user perspectives should all be taken into account in selection of how to measure an outcome concept.

## Choose outcomes wisely

In summary, there are a wide range of *process outcomes* (measures of knowledge use) to assess adherence to EBP and *evaluative outcomes* (measures of impact) to determine the effect of implementing EBP. The outcome examples presented in this chapter relate to the exemplar cases with chronic wounds (summarized in Table 5.1). They demonstrate the range of outcome choices, and the need for sensitivity in selecting specific outcomes for specific purposes. It is absolutely essential to consider the *user's perspective* and potential application of the outcome information: Does the outcome convince practitioners or decision makers or both? Is it for formative purposes to improve an implementation or summative purposes to demonstrate impact and inform health service choices about continuing with a particular approach?

Decision makers have to be willing (or convinced) to invest the necessary time and resources into monitoring and evaluation. In real world situations, data must be gathered in a timely manner and be clinically and administratively sensible and feasible. The evaluators must have the intellectual flexibility to use a full toolkit of methodologies in order to make decisions that will produce reliable and valid outcomes collected in a timely manner in consideration of pragmatic factors. Decisions typically have to be made in limited time frames not always amenable to large-scale research efforts. Lastly, the appropriateness of outcome selection and measurement may be complicated. It should be purposeful and carefully thought-out. For instance, in both the chronic wound examples an important practice outcome is healing. However this outcome concept can be measured in numerous ways, including 3-month rates, time-to-healing, wound size reduction, full-limb healing versus reference ulcer healing (usually designated as the largest ulcer), durability of healing (length of time ulcer free), and recurrence. Each of these methods has specific rigor, clinical sensibility, and feasibility characteristics that may influence the quality of completeness of the information gathered.

## Conclusion

Outcomes should be considered the linchpin in driving and sustaining EBP. Strategic selection of outcomes first and foremost contributes to accurate and useful monitoring of the uptake of evidence-based recommended care. It can be instrumental to informing quality and risk management processes and provides "local" evidence about the problem and the context. Secondly outcomes contribute to evaluating how care has improved through the use of evidence at the level of the patient, the provider, and the system. Lastly, outcomes developed throughout an implementation can provide evidence about the worth of sustaining EBPs.

## References

Agency for Healthcare Research and Quality (AHCPR) (1992). Preventing pressure ulcers: A patient's guide, AHCPR Publication No. 92-0048.

Bergstrom, N., Braden, B.J., Laguzza, A., & Holman, V. (1987). The Braden Scale for predicting pressure sore risk, *Nursing Research*, 36(4), 205–210.

Braden, B. (1987). A conceptual schema for the study of the etiology of pressure sores. *Rehabilitation Nursing*, 12(1), 8–16.

Fisher, A., Denis, N., Harrison, M.B., McNamee, M., Friedberg, E., & Wells, G. (1996). Quality management in skin care: Understanding the problem of pressure ulcers, *Canadian Journal of Quality in Health Care*, 13(1), 4–11.

Friedberg, E.H., Harrison, M.B., & Graham, I.D. (2002). Current home care expenditures for persons with leg ulcers. *Ostomy Wound Management*, 29(4), 186–192.

Girouard, K., Harrison, M.B., & Vandenkerkhof, E. (2008). The symptom of pain with pressure ulcers—what is the evidence? *Ostomy Wound Management*, 54(5), 30–42.

Graham, I.D., Lorimer, K., Harrison, M.B., & Pierscianowski, T. (2000). Evaluating the quality of international clinical practice guidelines for leg ulcers: Preparing for a Canadian adaptation. *Canadian Association of Enterostomal Therapy Journal*, 19(3), 15–31.

Graham, I.D., Harrison, M.B., Moffat, C., & Franks, P. (2001). Leg ulcer care: Nursing attitudes and knowledge. *Canadian Nurse*, 97(3), 19–24.

Graham, I.D., Harrison, M.B., Nelson, E.A., Lorimer, K., & Fisher, A. (2003a). Prevalence of lower-limb ulceration: A systematic review of prevalence studies, *Advances in Skin & Wound Care*, 16, 305–316.

Graham, I.D., Harrison, M.B., Shafey, M., & Keast, D. (2003b). Knowledge and attitudes regarding care of leg ulcers. *Canadian Family Physician*, 49, 896–920.

Graham, I.D., Harrison, M.B., Lorimer, K. et al. (2004). Adapting national and international leg ulcer practice guidelines for local use: The Ontario leg ulcer community care protocol. Implementing Evidence Based Practice in Nursing and Midwifery: A collection of papers presented at the Concurrent National Symposia, Joanna Briggs Institute, pp. 49–72.

Harrison, M.B. (2008). Pressure ulcer monitoring: A process of evidence-based practice, quality, and research. *Joint Commission Journal of Quality and Patient Safety*, 34(6), 355–359.

Harrison, M.B., Wells, G., Fisher, A., & Prince, M. (1996). Practice guidelines for the prediction and prevention of pressure ulcers: Evaluating the evidence. *Journal of Applied Nursing Research*, 9(1), 9–17.

Harrison, M.B., Logan, J., Joseph, L., & Graham, I.D. (1998). Quality improvement, research, and evidence-based practice: 5 years experience with pressure ulcers. *Evidence-based Nursing*, 1(4), 108–110.

Harrison, M.B., Nelson, E.A., Lorimer, K., Harris, C., & Vandenkerkhof, E. (2003). Community randomised control trial of the effectiveness of two compression bandaging technologies. *Canadian Institutes of Health Research (#MCT-63175)*, 2003–2009.

Harrison, M.B., Graham, I.D., Lorimer, K., Friedberg, E., Pierscianowski, T., & Brandys, T. (2005). Leg-ulcer care in the community, before and after implementation of an evidence-based service. *Canadian Medical Association Journal*, 172(11), 1447–1452.

Harrison, M.B., Graham, I., Lorimer, K. et al. 2008. Nurse clinic versus home delivery of community leg ulcer care: A Canadian Randomized Controlled Trial. *BMC Health Services Research*, 8, 243.

Logan, J., Harrison, M.B., Graham, I.D., Dunn, K., & Bissonnette, J. (1999). Evidence-based pressure ulcer practice: The Ottawa model of research use. *Canadian Journal of Nursing Research*, 31(1), 37–52.

Mackey, M., Draper, S., Harrison, M.B., & Friedberg, E. (2005). Possible contributing factors in pressure ulcer prevalence: A pilot study of two medical units. *Wound Care Canada*, 3(1), 38–40.

National Pressure Ulcer Advisory Panel (1989), Pressure ulcers: Prevalence, cost and risk assessment. Consensus development Conference Statement. *Decubitus*, 2(2), 24–28.

Nemeth, K.A., Graham, I.D., & Harrison, M.B. (2003a). The measurement of leg ulcer pain: Identification and appraisal of pain assessment tools. *Advances in Skin & Wound Care*, 16(5), 260–267.

Nemeth, K.A., Harrison, M.B., Graham, I.D., & Burke, S. (2003b). Pain in pure and mixed aetiology venous leg ulcers: A three-phase point prevalence study, *Journal of Wound Care*, 12(9), 336–340.

Vandenkerkhof, E., Harrison, M.B., & Friedberg, E. (2005). Prevalence of adverse events in acute care: Pressure ulcer risk & occurrence over ten years. *American Journal of Epidemiology*, 161S, S58.

# Chapter 6

# Implementing and sustaining evidence in nursing care of cardiovascular disease

*Anne Sales*

---

**Key learning points**

- Care for patients with cardiovascular disease is a rapidly evolving area in which new evidence is being generated constantly. Nurses and nursing interventions are among the forefront of efforts to improve the quality of care patients with cardiovascular disease experience.
- A number of different kinds of nursing interventions have evidence to support their usefulness in improving care to patients with cardiovascular disease. These include care pathways or critical care maps, case management, nurse-led clinics, and telehealth and e-health approaches.
- Outcomes used to measure effectiveness of improving quality of care for patients with cardiovascular disease range from "hard" outcomes like mortality and repeat hospitalizations to "soft" outcomes such as health-related quality of life. There are many different ways to measure health-related quality of life in cardiovascular disease.

- Despite the evidence of success of nursing interventions to improve quality of care and quality of life for patients with cardiovascular disease, substantial barriers remain to fully and effectively implementing these interventions. These include time and human resource constraints.

## Introduction

There are few clinical content areas in health care with more robust empirically based evidence than cardiovascular disease. Hundreds of randomized controlled trials (RCTs) have been conducted over many decades, leading to a very rich set of evidence-based guidelines and practice recommendations (cf. Antman et al. 2004; Krumholz et al. 2006; Schocken et al. 2008 among many others). This rich evidence base has led to a number of quality improvement efforts over many years in hospitals, outpatient centers, and other sites where care is delivered.

Despite this rich base of evidence generally available in cardiology, the majority of these guidelines focus on physician care. Most guidelines address use of devices and procedures, as well as medical management of patients experiencing both acute cardiovascular events and the effects of long-term, chronic disease. Few of these guidelines address non-physician care, although in some instances, recommendations are made for health care professionals other than physicians. This chapter will focus on the evidence for interventions that do not require physician action, although most of the clinical care provided to patients with cardiovascular disease includes multidisciplinary team care, and physicians are usually integral members of the health care team. Specific actions, such as ordering tests and procedures, prescribing medications, and ordering and/or delivering invasive procedures or placing devices into a patient's body, generally require at least physician oversight, and these will not be the major focus of this chapter, even though some of these actions can be performed by non-physician providers, such as advanced practice nurses and, in some jurisdictions, pharmacists. Other actions, including education, coaching, lifestyle modification approaches, monitoring and managing chronic disease (except for medication management), and working with patients in their homes and communities, are more often in the domain of nurses and other health care professionals, and I will focus on these activities.

In this chapter, I first provide an overview of cardiology and care for patients with cardiovascular disease, followed by a section describing specific care interventions that have substantial nursing input supported by research evidence. The focus here is to describe evidence-based practice (EBP) in nursing care for patients with cardiovascular disease. In the final section, I summarize the current impact of nursing-focused interventions for patients with cardiovascular disease.

## A brief history of the evolution of cardiology in practice

It is useful to review the profound changes in cardiovascular care driven by the emerging evidence base in cardiology. As recently as 40 years ago, there were few interventions available for people who experienced myocardial infarction (MI—death of heart muscle due to coronary artery disease, colloquially called a heart attack) (Malach & Imperato 2006). Patients either survived an MI, or died, and a high proportion died. Those who survived often experienced serious loss of heart muscle, which often led to serious compromise and the development of chronic heart failure. The only curative intervention available for coronary artery disease was coronary artery bypass grafting (CABG), in which a section of vein from the leg is grafted onto one or more coronary arteries to reopen the arteries. This was high-risk, expensive surgery, requiring that the chest wall be surgically opened to provide direct access to the coronary arteries. Only a limited number of hospitals had the capacity to perform it. This led to problems of access due to expense and geography. For many people with coronary artery disease, inability to pay or lack of physical access led to loss of heart muscle, loss of quality of life, and, in many cases, to early death.

In the intervening four decades, new approaches have revolutionized care for people with coronary artery disease, especially those with symptoms suggestive of coronary artery blockage. The most important were the advent of thrombolysis (Armstrong 2001), as well as percutaneous coronary intervention (PCI)—the use of minimally invasive methods to introduce balloons and stents (small metal strips that hold the artery open) through the vasculature into the coronary anatomy (Jamshidi et al. 2008; Melikian & Wijns 2008; Ryan et al. 2007); significant improvements in coronary artery bypass graft surgery, including improvements in anesthesia; the advent of drugs to lower blood cholesterol levels, particularly a class of drugs called statins, which not only lower blood cholesterol but also inhibit inflammation in the arteries (Schwartz 2007); and increasing evidence to show which drugs are most beneficial for patients with cardiovascular disease (Anderson et al. 2007; Bonow et al. 2008; Califf et al. 2007; Krumholz et al. 2008; Peterson et al. 2008). In the newest wave of evidence are findings that show that most patients with stable coronary artery disease can be managed medically, without invasive procedures of any kind (Boden & Gupta 2008; Boden et al. 2008; Eid & Boden 2008). However, there is also evidence that shows that a large proportion of patients who would benefit from medical management are not receiving optimal medical care, nor are they receiving invasive procedures. The picture is emerging of gaps related to gender, age, income, and possibly race and ethnicity, in providing evidence-based, individually optimized care (Austin et al. 2008; Ho et al. 2007; Jackevicius et al. 2008; Peterson et al. 2006; Pilote et al. 2007; Spertus & Furman 2007; Tricoci et al. 2007).

Most of these innovations were focused on care of patients with acute coronary syndromes (unstable angina or chest pain and MI), but they had ripple effects on care for other cardiovascular conditions. Important advances in care of heart failure and cardiac arrhythmias include implantable cardioverter defibrillators (Jung et al. 2008), and the use of new biomarkers for diagnosis and staging of heart failure (Andrade & Sharar 2008; McDonald et al. 2008). Biomarkers have also changed the approach to detecting and treating acute coronary syndromes and other cardiovascular disease (Abi-Saleh et al. 2008; Parikh & De Lemos 2006). Finally, yet more change is likely in the near future, as stem cell and genetic therapies offer new opportunities for diagnosis and treatment of cardiovascular disease (Anwaruddin et al. 2007; Eriksson et al. 2006; Hare & Chaparro 2008; Rahman & Maclellan 2006; Rizik et al. 2006). These changes were not only in procedures, devices, and drugs but they also motivated significant innovation in the systems of providing care to patients with cardiovascular disease.

## System approaches to changing delivery of cardiovascular care

The vast majority of procedures used to care for patients with acute coronary syndromes (over 90% in most developed countries) are now PCIs, rather than CABG. Rather than being performed in operating suites, PCI is performed in what are known as cardiac catheterization laboratories, or cardiac cath labs. Training for PCI is not a surgical specialty, but a sub-specialization within cardiology, which in turn is a sub-specialty of internal medicine or pediatrics. Although nurses and other professionals, including technicians, are trained to provide care within cardiac cath labs, care is quite different from surgery requiring general anesthesia; most cardiac catheterization and PCI procedures are done under conscious sedation. As a result, many procedures can be done on an ambulatory or outpatient basis, compared with the admissions required for CABG surgery. This innovation alone has revolutionized the care provided. Many hospitals have cardiac cath labs even though they do not have surgical suites. In general, if a hospital cannot provide CABG surgery as an emergency option, cardiac catheterization is limited to imaging, without providing reperfusion intervention such as PCI.

The movement to ambulatory care for patients who previously would have required surgery has led to other innovations in service delivery, including a renewed emphasis on secondary prevention, or attempting to ensure that someone who has suffered a previous episode of acute coronary syndrome does not experience another one. Secondary prevention is typically managed through primary care services in most countries, although it may be offered in the context of cardiac rehabilitation in others (Clark et al. 2005). Typically, cardiac rehabilitation focuses on lifestyle modification, as well as prescribing drugs that have been shown to decrease the risk of recurrent coronary and related events (MI, stroke, and death). Secondary prevention offered through primary care often focuses principally on drug prescribing and control of risk factors, including hypertension, diabetes, and renal disease. In primary care, this kind of secondary prevention is often described as chronic disease management or care, to emphasize the reality that the medications and/or lifestyle modification are required for the rest of the person's life, not just to assist during an acute episode (Balady et al. 2007; Thomas et al. 2007).

Nurses often provide frontline care in both cardiac rehabilitation and chronic disease management. In many places, nurses are the primary providers of secondary prevention or chronic disease management services; in others, they work collaboratively within a team of providers, who may include cardiologists, primary care physicians, dieticians, exercise physiologists, physical and occupational therapists, and other disciplines (Coons & Fera 2007). Nurses provide care in all settings, from emergency departments where initial emergent or urgent care is provided, to operative suites or cardiac cath labs, to coronary care or other inpatient acute care units, to outpatient ambulatory care either in primary care or rehabilitation. The rest of this chapter will focus on the evidence for the care that nurses provide for patients with cardiovascular disease.

## Outcomes and their impact

A wide variety of outcomes have been used to measure how well care is delivered (often called process outcomes), the extent to which care is related to desired outcomes (preference outcomes, including quality of life), and "hard" outcomes (Bonow et al. 2008; Mehta et al. 2007). The latter are usually a mixture of death, recurrent MI or unstable angina requiring hospitalization, or related events such as stroke. Among process outcomes, a number of outcomes have been proposed, and many are included in clinical practice guidelines as indicators of quality of care. These include measures such as:

- Administration of aspirin within 24 hours of onset of chest pain symptoms;
- Ensuring that all patients with documented MI are prescribed aspirin, beta-blockers, statins, and angiotensin-converting enzyme inhibitors (ACE-I), unless contraindicated, on hospital discharge (Ko et al. 2008).

More recently, health-related quality of life outcomes, related to patient preferences, have gained acceptance in cardiovascular care to assess the degree to which services and care provision affects how well people feel (Beinart et al. 2003; Rumsfeld et al. 2001, 2003). Health-related quality of life measures both perceived health status—how people feel—and preferences, which may include preferences about treatments, as well as preferences about the health state the person is in. Both disease-specific and generic health-related quality of life measures are used to measure outcomes of care (Spertus 2008; Spertus et al. 2008; Weintraub et al. 2008). Specific links to depression and other mental health issues have been noted for some time (Maddox et al. 2008; Plomondon et al. 2008; Sullivan et al. 2007).

All of these measures can be used to evaluate outcomes for providers other than physicians. For example, in a paper published several years ago, the relationship between nurse staffing on inpatient care units and in-hospital mortality for patients who had experienced an MI was examined, and an association between increased nurse staffing and lower rates of in-hospital death was found (Person et al. 2004). A number of nurse-specific interventions have been shown to improve quality indicators, or process outcomes, and nursing interventions have been shown to improve patient perception of quality of care.

The next section describes specific interventions in which nurses play a leading role in caring for patients with cardiovascular disease. Within each intervention type, I discuss specific cardiovascular health problems, and how the intervention applies to that health problem.

## Nursing-focused evidence-informed care for patients with cardiovascular health problems

### Care pathways or maps

Care pathways or care maps (also called critical or clinical pathways) are primarily used in inpatient care settings. They have been used extensively in care of patients with cardiovascular health problems, most often with patients suffering from chronic heart disease and acute coronary syndromes, although they have also been used in other cardiac conditions, such as syncope (Herzog et al. 2006). While this type of intervention has been around a long time, care pathways or maps are still being actively developed and implemented in inpatient care settings (Cannon 2008; Gardetto et al. 2008; Lombardo et al. 2008; de Luca et al. 2008; McDermott et al. 2008).

In general, care pathways are multidisciplinary guides that use evidence to develop protocols and specific steps for caring for patients from first contact with the hospital—often in the emergency department—through to hospital discharge. The most comprehensive approaches include specific protocols and instructions for discharge planning, and specify how and when patients should receive follow-up care. The types of care covered include medications to be used during hospitalization, and what should be prescribed at discharge, specific nursing interventions to assure that patients are progressing along a trajectory that will allow them to be discharged from the hospital and regain self-care function, and discharge instructions designed to minimize risk of rapid rehospitalization. Results from care pathways and maps are mixed, but when well designed and well implemented, they can result in considerable improvement (Gardetto et al. 2008).

The interdisciplinary aspect of care pathways or maps is essential. Full implementation requires the full collaboration of multiple disciplines (Peterson et al. 2008; Leggat 2007). Physicians are responsible for ensuring accurate diagnosis, staging, and prognosis, as well as for ordering appropriate tests and prescribing medications. Nurses are responsible for monitoring during the inpatient stay, ensuring that patients and families receive adequate and appropriate education to minimize risks, and managing discharge planning. This should include referrals to appropriate community agencies, as well as education about lifestyle and medication adherence.

A recent example of clinical path implementation describes how implementing a clinical path to manage acute decompensated heart failure during inpatient admission in a single academic health center resulted in more complete discharge instruction, and decreased readmissions to the hospital within 7 and 90 days after discharge (Lombardo et al. 2008). This is a fairly commonly reported result of implementing a clinical pathway. Most are locally derived and highly tailored to the specific hospital setting. The level of specificity often makes it difficult to move a developed clinical path from one hospital to another, as resources or even terms used to describe different roles may differ significantly from setting to setting.

In an attempt to deal with this problem, and to develop pathways that might transfer from one setting to another, there have been efforts to develop more generic toolkits to inform cardiac care that can be adapted from one hospital to another (Cannon et al. 2002; Mehta et al. 2002; Morrow & Cannon 2005). Some of these have focused on acute coronary syndromes, while others have focused on heart failure. Overall, these two cardiovascular health problems have been the greatest focus in clinical pathway development.

Early clinical pathways were not always as clear as they may have needed to be in delineating roles for each of the health care disciplines involved in providing care. Generally, if the pathway is not developed by an interdisciplinary team, it is difficult to ensure that appropriate roles and responsibilities are delineated. Even when roles and responsibilities are appropriate, there may be gaps in carrying out the actions required. One example, which crosses many different approaches to implementing EBP, is that nurses do not always have appropriate skills and knowledge to make community-based referrals (Edwards et al. 2007). In all likelihood, the members of the health care team with the best skills to manage referrals are social workers, but it is sometimes the case that their skills focus on referrals for social services rather than for health services. It is essential to give attention to issues such as referrals, and who among the team has the skills to manage them appropriately and efficiently. It may be necessary to expand the team as necessary competencies are mapped out through the care pathway development process.

In summary, clinical pathways are often good approaches to implementing clinical practice guidelines and EBP. The kinds of outcomes that have been studied include repeat hospitalization and mortality, but do not as yet include quality of life assessment. In order for clinical pathways to be effective, they must usually be tailored to local resources, and attention must be paid to specifying required roles and who will fulfill them. However, there is little evidence in the published, peer-reviewed literature about the sustainability of the results from implementing clinical pathways.

## Case management

Case management is a broad concept in which a health care professional is given responsibility for managing care of patients, usually a group of patients with similar health problems (Dougherty et al. 2000; Naylor et al. 1999, 2004; White & Hall 2006). For example, case management has been used extensively for patients with chronic heart failure (Sochalski et al. 2009). Generally, a single case manager is assigned to a group of patients (or caseload). Activity by case managers can range from daily follow-up (very intensive) to intermittent follow-up every 2–3 months. Most case managers follow their assigned patients by telephone, although sometimes they also use in-person visits, and increasingly, case management is supplemented by forms of telehealth or e-health. These will be discussed more in a later section, and in this section, I will focus on case management. It should be noted that terminology, which changes frequently in health care, appears to be evolving to use the term "disease management" often as a synonym for case management. Disease management is probably a somewhat broader topic, although it is often difficult to tell from published reports what elements beyond case management a specific disease management program offers.

Case management is often used in outpatient settings, and in transitions between one care setting and another. In particular, it has been used extensively in transitions from acute inpatient care to community or home care (McCauley et al. 2006; Naylor et al. 2004). In general, it has been shown to be effective in reducing hospital readmission, although it is most effective when patients are carefully selected or targeted for case management, rather than providing case management to patients who are able to manage their own care effectively. The services provided by case managers include follow-up telephone calls to checkup on patients and see how they are doing; consultation with physicians and other providers if the patient expresses problems; coordination of services, such as through an external agency; and, when needed, advice to seek urgent care, which may result in readmission to the hospital.

In a series of reports on a recently completed trial of nurse-led disease/case management, Sisk and colleagues (2006) describe significant benefits from case management of low-income patients with systolic heart failure. These included decreased hospitalization in the group that received the case management intervention, improved functional status, and improved health-related quality of life. In a companion piece evaluating cost-effectiveness, however, Hebert and colleagues (2008) make the point that the intervention was most cost-effective for the most seriously ill patients, those with Class IV heart failure. Further, Hebert and Sisk (2008) argue in a related commentary that it is difficult to assess which component of a complex intervention such as disease management, or case management, is actually producing an effect. It is almost impossible to distil out a "pure" form of case management, meaning that we do not know whether it is the regular contact, the trust relationship, the knowledge imparted during a telephone call, the support for dealing with problems and setbacks, or other aspects of the intervention that produce the effect.

In general, the literature on nurse case management or disease management suggests that it is relatively effective in enhancing patient adherence to guideline recommendations, both for medications and for lifestyle, but it is likely to be most effective with targeted patients who are either more severely ill, or who face challenges like poverty or health illiteracy. These interventions are seldom cost-effective when used with broad patient groups that mix patients with low- and high-disease severity together, and they are sometimes entirely ineffective without adequate targeting or selection of patients. Repeat hospitalizations are the most commonly measured outcomes for case management interventions.

## Nurse-led clinics

Nurse-led or nurse-directed clinics have been used fairly extensively for a variety of cardiovascular health problems (Bruggink-André De La Porte et al. 2007; Campbell et al. 1998; Koelewijn-Van Loon et al. 2008; McHugh et al. 2001; Murchie et al. 2003; Raftery et al. 2005). Nurse-led clinics take many forms, but should always include education and counseling provided by a nurse who is highly trained in the content of the clinic. Depending on the skill level and preparation of nurses in the clinic, nurse-led clinics may include prescribing and/or titrating medications to achieve therapeutic or optimal doses, or to minimize side effects. Sometimes nurse-led clinics include components provided by other types of health care professionals. Some clinics include both pharmacists and nurses, or nurses and exercise physiologists or kinesiologists. In the case of pharmacist/nurse clinics, pharmacists usually concentrate on issues related to medications and other therapeutic agents, while nurses focus on education, counseling, and coaching. In other interdisciplinary clinics, such as with exercise physiologists, the exercise physiologist would focus on exercise, physical function, and related lifestyle counseling and coaching, often including physical activity classes, while the nurse concentrates on other types of counseling, including medications.

In a study of nurse-led secondary prevention for coronary disease in Scotland, Campbell and colleagues evaluated the effects of a 1-year, nurse-led secondary prevention clinic at 1 year, 4 years, and 10 years (Campbell et al. 1998; Delaney et al. 2008; Murchie et al. 2003). They found that at 1 year, immediately following the initial intervention, patients randomized to the nurse-led clinic (compared to patients receiving usual primary care) had fewer deaths and fewer recurrent cardiac events. These gains were likely due to improved secondary prevention (use of aspirin, blood pressure management, lipid management, increased physical activity, and diet), although there was no difference between the two groups in smoking cessation (Campbell et al. 1998). After 4 years of follow-up, without further intervention, the improved mortality and decreased cardiac events persisted with significant differences between the two groups (Murchie et al. 2004). After 10 years of follow-up, the differences were no longer significant, although the mortality curves had not yet converged (Delaney et al. 2008). This is one of the longest follow-up periods of any trial of a nurse-led clinic, and it suggests that the gains from a 1-year intervention persist for some period of time. In a related cost-effectiveness analysis, costs of the nurse-led clinic intervention were higher for patients who received the nurse-led clinic intervention, although on average their total costs were slightly lower (not significantly different from the usual care control group) (Raftery et al. 2005). The nurse-led clinic intervention was found to be cost-effective using standard rules for judging cost-effectiveness of an intervention, due to the decreased number of deaths in the intervention group. Finally, the study investigators conducted a qualitative study of key staff who had been involved in the nurse-led clinics during the intervention period; the qualitative study was conducted at the same time as the 4-year follow-up study (Murchie et al. 2005). They found that most of the clinics that participated in the original RCT of the 1-year intervention had stopped the nurse-led clinics—although some had restarted them—despite the benefits the trial had shown. A number of factors were cited as barriers to continuing the clinics. The most prevalent of these were lack of resources, difficulty hiring staff, and problems with maintaining the teams over time. These are common problems associated with most nurse-focused interventions, and may reflect the realities of human resource constraints, as well as hierarchies within health care. As nurses take on roles that traditionally have been filled by physicians, when resources are scarce, these roles are among the first to be lost. This does not mean, however, that physicians have the time or capacity to take the roles up themselves, and so they are often simply unfilled under times of economic or other stress.

As with other interventions discussed, a nurse-led clinic may offer many different kinds of activities and interventions. Precisely which of these is effective, when there is an overall effect, may not be clear. As with other interventions, repeat hospitalization and mortality are common outcome measures.

## Telehealth and e-health

Telehealth and e-health (electronic methods of providing services) represent fast-growing new trends in health services delivery, and they have been quite extensively used as methods of extending the reach of health care professionals to provide cardiovascular care (Botsis & Hartvigsen 2008; Brunetti et al. 2008; Dellifraine & Dansky 2008; Fursse et al. 2008; Wakefield et al. 2008; Vasquez 2008). The most basic form of telehealth is monitoring a patient's condition by telephone, which is used extensively and has been used for decades. The innovation in telehealth and telecare is to systematize this monitoring, target patients who can benefit from it the most, and use it in place of in-person visits. Extensions of this basic service include interactive voice response telephone calls; use of home-based devices that can transmit blood pressure, pulse, ECG, and other vital status indicators, often including questions about weight gain, health status, and current concerns; videomonitoring using videophones or web-based systems such as webcams; and fully web-based systems for checking on current status. These latter innovations, when web-based technologies are used, are usually described as e-health. All of these types of innovations require human monitoring at some frequency. If a live health care professional is not involved in initiating contact with the patient and engaging in live, synchronous interaction, then periodic asynchronous monitoring must take place, with appropriate alerts to physicians, pharmacists, and other team members if there is evidence of physical deterioration or instability. Nurses usually provide the monitoring service, which extends the reach of the nurse beyond in-person physical presence, such as in an inpatient hospital unit, clinic, or nursing home. Ultimately, the expectation of these innovations is that patients can remain at home with adequate monitoring and remote intervention (such as advice to change medication dose, begin or stop a medication, or engage in a specific activity such as exercise), rather than require in-person visits either to the home by a health care professional, or to a clinic, hospital, or other health care facility by the patient.

Evidence on the effectiveness of these types of interventions is mixed. Recent studies of telehealth interventions among patients with heart failure generally show little effect of home telemonitoring. In a trial comparing the effect of home videomonitoring compared to home telephone monitoring compared to control patients with heart failure, Wakefield and colleagues (2008) found no evidence of benefit to videomonitoring over telephone monitoring, although when both intervention groups were combined, rates of readmission were lower for the intervention than control group. There were no statistically significant differences in mortality among the three groups. Disease-specific quality of life scores, measured by the Minnesota Living with Heart Failure questionnaire, were not significantly different among the three groups, although all three groups' scores improved over the period of the intervention. Similarly, Woodend and colleagues (2008) found that patients with heart failure who had home telemonitoring consisting of daily weight and blood pressure transmission, periodic ECG transmission, and weekly video-conferences with a nurse, which were mostly focused on education, had no differences in hospital readmission during follow-up, and only small differences among intervention and control group in quality of life scores. As in the Wakefield study (Wakefield et al. 2008), quality of life scores improved for both intervention and control groups over the study period.

By contrast, the patients with angina in the study by Woodend and colleagues (2008) had significantly lower hospital readmissions over the study period, and they had improvements in all of the Seattle Angina Questionnaire subscales. In a large trial of a telemonitoring intervention with patients with coronary artery disease, Waldman and colleagues (2008) found no difference between intervention and control patients in a composite end point which combined hospital readmission, recurrent events, and death, using an intent-to-treat analysis in which they analyzed all patients in the group to which they were assigned. However, when they analyzed whether patients in the intervention group actually used the telemonitoring system, they found that only 23% of patients randomized to intervention actually used the telemonitoring system. Differences in outcomes between patients who did and did not use the system, among the intervention group, were significant.

Dellifraine and Dansky (2008) conducted a recent systematic review and meta-analysis of telehealth care intervention in which they found that effectiveness overall is moderate, but positive. However, they found that the type of disease affects whether or not the intervention is effective, as do age of patients, gender, race/ethnicity, and specifics of the intervention. In their analysis, which included many different types of disease across several different studies, they found that telehealth interventions were more likely to be effective for heart disease than for diabetes, but they did not analyze whether effectiveness differed by type of heart disease.

In another review of telehealth intervention studies, Botsis and Hartvigsen (2008) found that a variety of issues affected the studies, ranging from issues of patient or provider acceptance and use of the telehealth intervention, to issues of organizational changes required to make the interventions functional. Similarly, in an exploratory study, Nahm and colleagues (2008) found that elderly patients given the option of using a telehealth monitoring system had multiple concerns. Most had web access, but many were unsure of how they might use computers to access the web for health care consultation. The most prevalent barrier was lack of self-efficacy in understanding health information, and concern that they would not be able to understand interventions and information they might receive.

All of these studies point to recurring themes in innovations to improve quality of care delivered to patients with cardiovascular disease. It is important to assess patients' fit with the innovation, especially if a technologically sophisticated or potentially challenging technology is being considered, and it is critical to carefully select or target patients who are most likely to benefit from intervention and higher levels of attention.

## Conclusion

A number of innovative methods have been developed and tested in which nurses can play an important role to implement and sustain EBP when providing care to patients with cardiovascular disease. These methods cross settings, although the majority are focused on outpatient care. This makes sense, as the two major reasons for implementing these innovations are to improve quality of care and outcomes for patients with cardiovascular disease, and also to decrease costs and utilization of expensive health care services, particularly hospitalization. These innovations have mixed effectiveness, and most suffer from some problems of implementation.

Frequent causes of problems in implementation are changes in roles, responsibilities, and delivery systems, among health care professionals and patients (and their families). Many of these innovations require either standing protocols or expanded roles of non-physician health care professionals, particularly nurses, or marked devolution of professional responsibility and control for managing care from professionals to patients and families. Both raise difficulties in terms of current systems of care, medicolegal liability issues, and professional relationships. It is likely that economic pressures, including the aging of the population with its attendant needs and demands for health services, and current economic stressors, will force and sustain changes in the health care system. Innovations such as these described here may offer some opportunities for cost-effective care.

None of these innovations represent panaceas. Recurring themes include the need for explicit targeting of patients who are most likely to benefit from implementing the innovation: the sickest, poorest, and most disadvantaged patients are the most likely to derive benefit. Other recurring themes include the need to adequately prepare both providers and patients with knowledge, tools and resources to deploy the innovation appropriately and provide technical support when needed. These are likely to be especially important with novel technologies such as high-end telemonitoring and e-health innovations. This kind of support will increase costs, at least in the short run, but over the long run, if the innovations are strengthened and institutionalized, may result in lowering overall costs for health care systems and possibly for society.

Another important point is that focusing solely on "hard" outcomes—mortality, rehospitalization, service utilization—may obscure significant gains in quality of life and other markers of quality of care. The most common finding of studies of innovations in health care delivery is that the innovation is not significantly better than usual care in reducing hard outcomes. Innovations in delivery are seldom worse than usual care. Ignoring possible improvements in outcomes such as quality of life and functional status may provide an argument for maintaining usual care as the status quo, despite the fact that usual care is not significantly better than the innovation. Costs are seldom measured, and if they are, seldom amortized over time appropriately to evaluate how important one-time costs are over the period of benefit. For some, the arguments for the status quo seem compelling, but this is largely in the face of little knowledge of true costs and perhaps more subtle and important outcomes. We are certainly in a much better position to measure outcomes related to quality of life, functional, and health status than at any time in the past, and our understanding of these outcomes is likely to drive decision making about how best to deliver services into the future, as more studies incorporate these outcomes into their design. In the literature reviewed for this chapter, studies published after 2006 were more likely to include quality of life outcomes than studies published before 2006.

Cardiology and care for people with cardiovascular health problems remains an area of innovation and experimentation. While there are still challenges, there are many opportunities for innovative practice and service delivery over the next several decades.

# References

Abi-Saleh, B., Iskandar, S.B., Elgharib, N., & Cohen, M.V. (2008). C-reactive protein: The harbinger of cardiovascular diseases. *Southern Medical Journal*, 101(5), 525–533.

Anderson, J.L., Adams, C.D., Antman, E.M. et al. (2007). ACC/AHA 2007 guidelines for the management of patients with unstable angina/non ST-elevation myocardial infarction: a report of the American College of Cardiology/American Heart Association Task Force on Practice Guidelines (Writing Committee to Revise the 2002 Guidelines for the Management of Patients With Unstable Angina/Non ST-Elevation Myocardial Infarction), *Circulation*, 116, 7.

Andrade, A. & Sharar, H. (2008). Natriuretic peptides: Putting the evidence into practice. *Canadian Journal of Cardiovascular Nursing (Journal canadien en soins infirmiers cardiovasculaires)*, 18(4), 34–39.

Antman, E.M., Anbe, D.T., Armstrong, P.W. et al. (2004). ACC/AHA guidelines for the management of patients with ST-elevation myocardial infarction: A report of the American College of Cardiology/American Heart Association Task Force on Practice Guidelines (Committee to Revise the 1999 Guidelines for the Management of patients with acute myocardial infarction), *Journal of the American College of Cardiology*, 44(3), E1–E211.

Anwaruddin, S., Askari, A.T., & Topol, E.J. (2007). Redefining risk in acute coronary syndromes using molecular medicine. *Journal of the American College of Cardiology*, 49(3), 279–289.

Armstrong, P.W. (2001). New advances in the management of acute coronary syndromes: 2. Fibrinolytic therapy for acute ST-segment elevation myocardial infarction. *Canadian Medical Association Journal*, 165(6), 791–797.

Austin, P.C., Tu, J.V., Ko, D.T., & Alter, D.A. (2008). Factors associated with the use of evidence-based therapies after discharge among elderly patients with myocardial infarction. *Canadian Medical Association Journal*, 179(9), 901–908.

Balady, G.J., Williams, M.A., Ades, P.A. et al. (2007). Core components of cardiac rehabilitation/secondary prevention programs: 2007 Update—A scientific statement from the American Heart Association Exercise, Cardiac Rehabilitation, and Prevention Committee, the Council on Clinical Cardiology; the Councils on Cardiovascular Nursing, Epidemiology and Prevention, and Nutrition, Physical Activity, and Metabolism. *Journal of Cardiopulmonary Rehabilitation and Prevention*, 27(3), 121–129.

Beinart, S.C., Sales, A.E., Spertus, J.A., Plomondon, M.E., Every, N.R., & Rumsfeld, J.S. (2003). Impact of angina burden and other factors on treatment satisfaction after acute coronary syndromes. *American Heart Journal*, 146(4), 646–652.

Boden, W.E. & Gupta, V. (2008). Reperfusion strategies in acute ST-segment elevation myocardial infarction. *Current Opinion in Cardiology*, 23(6), 613–619.

Boden, W.E., Shah, P.K., Gupta, V., & Ohman, E.M. (2008). Contemporary approach to the diagnosis and management of non-ST-segment elevation acute coronary syndromes. *Progress in Cardiovascular Diseases*, 50(5), 311–351.

Bonow, R.O., Masoudi, F.A., Rumsfeld, J.S. et al. (2008). ACC/AHA classification of care metrics: Performance measures and quality metrics—A report of the American College of Cardiology/American Heart Association Task Force on Performance Measures. *Circulation*, 118(24), 2662–2666.

Botsis, T. & Hartvigsen, G. (2008). Current status and future perspectives in telecare for elderly people suffering from chronic diseases. *Journal of Telemedicine and Telecare*, 14(4), 195–203.

Bruggink-André De La Porte, P.W.F., Lok, D.J.A., Van Veldhuisen, D.J. et al. (2007). Added value of a physician-and-nurse-directed heart failure clinic: Results from the Deventer-Alkmaar heart failure study. *Heart*, 93(7), 819–825.

Brunetti, N.D., Amodio, G., De Gennaro, L. et al. (2008). Telecardiology applied to a region-wide public emergency health-care service. *Journal of Thrombosis and Thrombolysis*, 1–8.

Califf, R.M., Mehta, R.H., & Peterson, E.D. (2007). Clinical quality in non-ST-elevation acute coronary syndromes. *American Journal of Medicine*, 120(11), 930–935.

Campbell, N.C., Ritchie, L.D., Thain, J., Deans, H.G., Rawles, J.M., & Squair, J.L. (1998). Secondary prevention in coronary heart disease: A randomised trial of nurse led clinics in primary care. *Heart*, 80(5), 447–452.

Cannon, C.P. (2008). Updated strategies and therapies for reducing ischemic and vascular events (STRIVE) ST-segment elevation myocardial infarction critical pathway toolkit. *Critical Pathways in Cardiology*, 7(4), 223–231.

Cannon, C.P., Hand, M.H., Bahr, R. et al. (2002). Critical pathways for management of patients with acute coronary syndromes: An assessment by the National Heart Attack Alert Program. *American Heart Journal*, 143(5), 777–789.

Clark, A.M., Hartling, L., Vandermeer, B., & McAlister, F.A. (2005). Meta-analysis: Secondary prevention programs for patients with coronary artery disease. *Annals of Internal Medicine*, 143(9), 659–672.

Coons, J.C. & Fera, T. (2007). Multidisciplinary team for enhancing care for patients with acute myocardial infarction or heart failure. *American Journal of Health-System Pharmacy*, 64(12), 1274–1278.

Delaney, E.K., Murchie, P., Lee, A.J., Ritchie, L.D., & Campbell, N.C. (2008). Secondary prevention clinics for coronary heart disease: A 10-year follow-up of a randomised controlled trial in primary care. *Heart*, 94(11), 1419–1423.

Dellifraine, J.L. & Dansky, K.H. (2008). Home-based telehealth: A review and meta-analysis. *Journal of Telemedicine and Telecare*, 14(2), 62–66.

Dougherty, C.M., Spertus, J.A., Dewhurst, T.A., & Nichol, W.P. (2000). Outpatient nursing case management for cardiovascular disease. *The Nursing Clinics of North America*, 35(4), 993–1003.

Edwards, N., Davies, B., Ploeg, J., Virani, T., & Skelly, J. (2007). Implementing nursing best practice guidelines: Impact on patient referrals. *BMC Nursing*, 6, 4.

Eid, F. & Boden, W.E. (2008). The evolving role of medical therapy for chronic stable angina. *Current Cardiology Reports*, 10(4), 263–271.

Eriksson, S., Wittfooth, S., & Pettersson, K. (2006). Present and future biochemical markers for detection of acute coronary syndrome. *Critical Reviews in Clinical Laboratory Sciences*, 43(5–6), 427–495.

Fursse, J., Clarke, M., Jones, R., Khemka, S., & Findlay, G. (2008). Early experience in using telemonitoring for the management of chronic disease in primary care. *Journal of Telemedicine and Telecare*, 14(3), 122–124.

Gardetto, N.J., Greaney, K., Arai, L. et al. (2008). Critical pathway for the management of acute heart failure at the Veterans Affairs San Diego Healthcare System: Transforming performance measures into cardiac care. *Critical Pathways in Cardiology*, 7(3), 153–172.

Hare, J.M. & Chaparro, S.V. (2008). Cardiac regeneration and stem cell therapy. *Current Opinion in Organ Transplantation*, 13(5), 536–542.

Hebert, P.L. & Sisk, J.E. (2008). Challenges facing nurse-led disease management for heart failure. *Disease Management and Health Outcomes*, 16(1), 1–6.

Hebert, P.L., Sisk, J.E., Wang, J.J. et al. (2008). Cost-effectiveness of nurse-led disease management for heart failure in an ethnically diverse urban community. *Annals of Internal Medicine*, 149(8), 540–548.

Herzog, E., Frankenberger, O., Pierce, W., & Steinberg, J.S. (2006). The SELF pathway for the management of syncope. *Critical Pathways in Cardiology*, 5(3), 173–178.

Ho, P.M., Luther, S.A., Masoudi, F.A. et al. (2007). Inpatient and follow-up cardiology care and mortality for acute coronary syndrome patients in the Veterans Health Administration. *American Heart Journal*, 154(3), 489–494.

Jackevicius, C.A., Li, P., & Tu, J.V. (2008). Prevalence, predictors, and outcomes of primary nonadherence after acute myocardial infarction. *Circulation*, 117(8), 1028–1036.

Jamshidi, P., Mahmoody, K., & Erne, P. (2008). Covered stents: A review. *International Journal of Cardiology*, 130(3), 310–318.

Jung, W., Rillig, A., Birkemeyer, R., Miljak, T., & Meyerfeldt, U. (2008). Advances in remote monitoring of implantable pacemakers, cardioverter defibrillators and cardiac resynchronization therapy systems. *Journal of Interventional Cardiac Electrophysiology*, 23(1), 73–85.

Ko, D.T., Wijeysundera, H.C., Zhu, X. et al. (2008). Canadian quality indicators for percutaneous coronary interventions. *Canadian Journal of Cardiology*, 24(12), 899–903.

Koelewijn-Van Loon, M.S., Van Steenkiste, B., Ronda, G. et al. (2008). Improving patient adherence to lifestyle advice (IMPALA): A cluster-randomised controlled trial on the implementation of a nurse-led intervention for cardiovascular risk management in primary care (protocol). *BMC Health Services Research*, 8, 9.

Krumholz, H.M., Anderson, J.L., Brooks, N.H. et al. (2006). ACC/AHA clinical performance measures for adults with ST-elevation and non-ST-elevation myocardial infarction: A report of the American College of Cardiology/American Heart Association Task Force on Performance Measures (Writing committee to develop performance measures on ST-elevation and non-ST-elevation myocardial infarction). *Circulation*, 113(5), 732–761.

Krumholz, H.M., Anderson, J.L., Bachelder, B.L. et al. (2008). ACC/AHA 2008 performance measures for adults with ST-elevation and non-ST-elevation myocardial infarction: A report of the American College of Cardiology/American Heart Association Task Force on Performance Measures (Writing committee to develop performance measures for ST-elevation and non-ST-elevation myocardial infarction). *Circulation*, 118(24), 2596–2648.

Leggat, S.G. (2007). Effective healthcare teams require effective team members: Defining teamwork competencies. *BMC Health Services Research*, 7, 17.

Lombardo, D., Bridgeman, T.V., De Michelis, N., & Nunez, M. (2008). An academic medical centre's programme to develop clinical pathways to manage health care: Focus on acute decompensated heart failure. *Journal of Integrated Care Pathways*, 12(2), 45–55.

de Luca, A., Gabriele, S., Lauria, L. et al. (2008). Implementation of an emergency clinical pathway for ST-elevation myocardial infarction in the Lazio Region: Results of a pilot study. *Giornale Italiano di Cardiologia*, 9, 118–125.

Maddox, T.M., Reid, K.J., Spertus, J.A. et al. (2008). Angina at 1 year after myocardial infarction: Prevalence and associated findings. *Archives of Internal Medicine*, 168(12), 1310–1316.

Malach, M. & Imperato, P.J. (2006). Acute myocardial infarction and acute coronary syndrome: Then and now (1950–2005). *Preventive Cardiology*, 9(4), 228–234.

McCauley, K.M., Bixby, M.B. & Naylor, M.D. (2006). Advanced practice nurse strategies to improve outcomes and reduce cost in elders with heart failure. *Disease Management*, 9(5), 302–310.

McDermott, K.A., Helfrich, C.D., Sales, A.E., Rumsfeld, J.S., Ho, P.M. & Fihn, S.D. (2008). A review of interventions and system changes to improve time to reperfusion for ST-segment elevation myocardial infarction. *Journal of General Internal Medicine*, 23(8), 1246–1256.

McDonald, K., Dahlström, U., Aspromonte, N. et al. (2008). B-type natriuretic peptide: Application in the community. *Congestive Heart Failure (Greenwich, Conn.)*, 14(4 Suppl. 1), 12–16.

McHugh, F., Lindsay, G.M., Hanlon, P. et al. (2001). Nurse led shared care for patients on the waiting list for coronary artery bypass surgery: A randomised controlled trial. *Heart*, 86(3), 317–323.

Mehta, R.H., Montoye, C.K., Gallogly, M. et al. (2002). Improving quality of care for acute myocardial infarction: The Guidelines Applied in Practice (GAP) Initiative. *JAMA: The Journal of the American Medical Association*, 287(10), 1269–1276.

Mehta, R.H., Peterson, E.D., & Califf, R.M. (2007). Performance measures have a major effect on cardiovascular outcomes: A review. *The American Journal of Medicine*, 120(5), 398–402.

Melikian, N. & Wijns, W. (2008). Drug-eluting stents: A critique. *Heart*, 94(2), 145–152.

Morrow, D.A. & Cannon, C.P. (2005). Brigham and Women's Hospital admission order set for unstable angina/non-ST elevation myocardial infarction. *Critical Pathways in Cardiology*, 4(2), 107–109.

Murchie, P., Campbell, N.C., Ritchie, L.D., & Robson, J. (2003). Nurse led disease management clinics may improve long-term coronary heart disease outcomes in primary care. *Evidence-Based Healthcare*, 7(2), 55–56.

Murchie, P., Campbell, N.C., Ritchie, L.D., Deans, H.G., & Thain, J. (2004). Effects of secondary prevention clinics on health status in patients with coronary heart disease: 4 year follow-up of a randomized trial in primary care. *Family Practice*, 21(5), 567–574.

Murchie, P., Campbell, N.C., Ritchie, L.D., & Thain, J. (2005). Running nurse-led secondary prevention clinics for coronary heart disease in primary care: Qualitative study of health professionals' perspectives. *British Journal of General Practice*, 55(516), 522–528.

Nahm, E.S., Blum, K., Scharf, B. et al. (2008). Exploration of patients' readiness for an eHealth management program for chronic heart failure: A preliminary study. *Journal of Cardiovascular Nursing*, 23(6), 463–471.

Naylor, M.D., Brooten, D., Campbell, R. et al. (1999). Comprehensive discharge planning and home follow-up of hospitalized elders: A randomized clinical trial. *Journal of the American Medical Association*, 281(7), 613–620.

Naylor, M.D., Brooten, D.A., Campbell, R.L., Maislin, G., McCauley, K.M., & Schwartz, J.S. (2004). Transitional care of older adults hospitalized with heart failure: A randomized, controlled trial. *Journal of the American Geriatrics Society*, 52(5), 675–684.

Parikh, S.V. & De Lemos, J.A. (2006). Biomarkers in cardiovascular disease: Integrating pathophysiology into clinical practice. *American Journal of the Medical Sciences*, 332(4), 186–197.

Person, S.D., Allison, J.J., Kiefe, C.I. et al. (2004). Nurse staffing and mortality for medicare patients with acute myocardial infarction. *Medical Care*, 42(1), 4–12.

Peterson, E.D., Roe, M.T., Mulgund, J. et al. (2006). Association between hospital process performance and outcomes among patients with acute coronary syndromes. *JAMA: The Journal of the American Medical Association*, 295(16), 1912–1920.

Peterson, E.D., Albert, N.M., Amin, A., Patterson, J.H., & Fonarow, G.C. (2008). Implementing critical pathways and a multidisciplinary team approach to cardiovascular disease management. *American Journal of Cardiology*, 102(Suppl. 5), 47–56.

Pilote, L., Tu, J.V., Humphries, K. et al. (2007). Socioeconomic status, access to health care, and outcomes after acute myocardial infarction in Canada universal health care system. *Medical Care*, 45(7), 638–646.

Plomondon, M.E., Magid, D.J., Masoudi, F.A. et al. (2008). Association between angina and treatment satisfaction after myocardial infarction. *Journal of General Internal Medicine*, 23(1), 1–6.

Raftery, J.P., Yao, G.L., Murchie, P., Campbell, N.C., & Ritchie, L.D. (2005). Cost effectiveness of nurse led secondary prevention clinics for coronary heart disease in primary care: Follow up of a randomised controlled trial. *British Medical Journal*, 330(7493), 707–710.

Rahman, J.E. & Maclellan, W.R. (2006). Fundamentals of stem cell mobilization for the heart: Prospects for treating heart disease. *Current Opinion in Investigational Drugs*, 7(9), 799–805.

Rizik, D.G., Klassen, K.J., Dowler, D.A., Villegas, B.J., & Dixon, S.R. (2006). Promising though not yet proven: Emerging strategies to promote myocardial salvage. *Catheterization and Cardiovascular Interventions*, 68(4), 596–606.

Rumsfeld, J.S., Magid, D.J., Plomondon, M.E. et al. (2001). Predictors of quality of life following acute coronary syndromes. *The American Journal of Cardiology*, 88(7), pp. 781–784.

Rumsfeld, J.S., Magid, D.J., Plomondon, M.E. et al. (2003). History of depression, angina, and quality of life after acute coronary syndromes. *American Heart Journal*, 145(3), 493–499.

Ryan, J., Cutlip, D.E., Cohen, D.J., & Pinto, D.S. (2007). Drug eluting stents for ST-elevation myocardial infarction: Risk and benefit. *Journal of Thrombosis and Thrombolysis*, 24(3), 293–299.

Schocken, D.D., Benjamin, E.J., Fonarow, G.C. et al. (2008) Prevention of heart failure: A scientific statement from the American Heart Association Councils on epidemiology and prevention, clinical cardiology, cardiovascular nursing, and high blood pressure research; Quality of Care and Outcomes Research Interdisciplinary Working Group; and Functional Genomics and Translational Biology Interdisciplinary Working Group. *Circulation*, 117(19), 2544–2565.

Schwartz, G.G. (2007). Lipid management after acute coronary syndrome. *Current Opinion in Lipidology*, 18(6), 626–632.

Sisk, J.E., Hebert, P.L., Horowitz, C.R., McLaughlin, M.A., Wang, J.J., & Chassin, M.R. (2006). Effects of nurse management on the quality of heart failure care in minority communities: A randomized trial. *Annals of Internal Medicine*, 145(4), 273–283.

Sochalski, J., Jaarsma, T., Krumholz, H.M. et al. (2009). What works in chronic care management: The case of heart failure. *Health Affairs*, 28(1), 179–189.

Spertus, J.A. (2008). Evolving applications for patient-centered health status measures. *Circulation*, 118(20), 2103–2110.

Spertus, J.A. & Furman, M.I. (2007). Translating evidence into practice: Are we neglecting the neediest? *Archives of Internal Medicine*, 167(10), 987–988.

Spertus, J.A., Jones, P.G., Kim, J., & Globe, D. (2008). Validity, reliability, and responsiveness of the Kansas City Cardiomyopathy Questionnaire in anemic heart failure patients. *Quality of Life Research*, 17(2), 291–298.

Sullivan, M.D., Levy, W.C., Russo, J.E., Crane, B., & Spertus, J.A. (2007). Summary health status measures in advanced heart failure: Relationship to clinical variables and outcome. *Journal of Cardiac Failure*, 13(7), 560–568.

Thomas, R.J., King, M., Lui, K. et al. (2007). AACVPR/ACC/AHA 2007 performance measures on cardiac rehabilitation for referral to and delivery of cardiac rehabilitation/secondary prevention services. Endorsed by the American College of Chest Physicians, American College of Sports Medicine, American Physical Therapy Association, Canadian Association of Cardiac Rehabilitation, European Association for Cardiovascular.... *Journal of the American College of Cardiology*, 50(14), 1400–1433.

Tricoci, P., Peterson, E.D., Chen, A.Y. et al. (2007). Timing of glycoprotein IIb/IIIa inhibitor use and outcomes among patients with non-ST-segment elevation myocardial infarction undergoing percutaneous coronary intervention (Results from CRUSADE). *The American Journal of Cardiology*, 99(10), 1389–1393.

Vasquez, M.S. (2008). Down to the fundamentals of telehealth and home healthcare nursing. *Home Healthcare Nurse*, 26(5), 280–287.

Wakefield, B.J., Ward, M.M., Holman, J.E. et al. (2008). Evaluation of home telehealth following hospitalization for heart failure: A randomized trial. *Telemedicine and e-Health*, 14(8), 753–761.

Waldmann, A., Katalinic, A., Schwaab, B., Richardt, G., Sheikhzadeh, A., & Raspe, H. (2008). The TeleGuard trial of additional telemedicine care in CAD patients. 2 Morbidity and mortality after 12 months. *Journal of Telemedicine and Telecare*, 14(1), 22–26.

Weintraub, W.S., Spertus, J.A., Kolm, P. et al. (2008). Effect of PCI on quality of life in patients with stable coronary disease. *New England Journal of Medicine*, 359(7), 677–687.

White, P. & Hall, M.E. (2006). Mapping the literature of case management nursing. *Journal of the Medical Library Association*, 94(Suppl. 2), E99–E106.

Woodend, A.K., Sherrard, H., Fraser, M., Stuewe, L., Cheung, T., & Struthers, C. (2008). Telehome monitoring in patients with cardiac disease who are at high risk of readmission. *Heart and Lung: Journal of Acute and Critical Care*, 37(1), 36–45.

# Chapter 7

# Outcomes of implementation that matter to health service users

*Debra Bick and Ian D. Graham*

**Key learning points**

- There is increased recognition that the involvement of service users in the design, content, and evaluation of health service provision is essential to achieve and sustain high-quality health care.
- Service user involvement in all stages of the research process is now also viewed as essential. Many funding agencies require that service users are equal partners in funding bids.
- Evidence of the impact of greater involvement of service users in the planning, development, and dissemination of national policy and research priorities is evolving.
- The outcomes of evidence-based practice (EBP) from a service user perspective can reflect a spectrum of involvement from representation on an advisory group, involvement in decisions about day-to-day care or a decision to participate in a research study.
- There is an extensive and developing evidence base that describes how many different studies have involved service users.

## Introduction

There has been increasing recognition over recent years that the involvement of health service users and their families, private and voluntary sectors, and wider public in the design, content, and delivery of health services is essential to achieve and sustain high-quality care. In parallel, users have become increasingly involved in different stages of the research process to inform findings which are relevant and appropriate for users (Staniszewska et al. 2007; Tarpey 2006 ). In some areas of health-care provision, most noticeably maternity care, there is a long history of the direct involvement of service users in the questioning of practice and policy, often as a consequence of views which differed markedly from accepted "best" practice at the time. An example of this was the widespread use of routine episiotomy in UK maternity care during the 1970s, which was purported by clinicians to have a number of advantages over restricted use, an assumed benefit questioned by women. Evidence from large randomized controlled trials (RCTs) which compared outcomes of restrictive with routine episiotomy showed no benefit from routine use (Carroli & Mignini 2008). Although change in practice in the UK and other English-speaking countries appears to have commenced prior to the publication of trial findings, this does not detract from the challenge study findings presented to the beliefs of maternity providers (Graham et al. 2005). That routine episiotomy persists in many developed and developing countries appears to be a consequence of health-care providers' beliefs about the value of the procedure and women's inability to give birth without surgical intervention (Graham 1996). It is also possibly because user involvement is not as widespread or proactive in these countries and because care is dominated by a medical model. This highlights the levels of complexity and influence of culture, context, and individual belief systems relating to use of evidence-based practice (EBP) and why harmful health practices persist while potentially beneficial practices are not universally implemented (McGlynn et al. 2003; Schuster et al. 1998).

As referred to in Chapter 2, EBP is a type of knowledge use, primarily knowledge derived from research, the outcomes from which can be divided into two broad categories: knowledge use and its impact. This chapter will outline the recent focus on service user involvement in determining the outcomes of EBP, initiatives to increase their contribution to health service policy and research and how their experiences of care are being captured and disseminated (the term *service user* is used throughout this chapter to include patients, their immediate carers outside of health-care professionals, and other commonly used terms such as health consumers). As this is a relatively new area, service user perspectives have not been reflected in the development of models and frameworks to support EBP although this situation is likely to change (Graham et al. 2006).

## Enhancing the contribution of service users to health service policy and research

### The role of national agencies

In the UK there was a noticeable shift in health service policy and research priority setting following the election of a Labour government in 1997 from a position of managing ill-health to a position of *prevention* of ill-health, including the need for individuals to take greater responsibility for their own health (Department of Health 1999). Although the success of this approach when viewed a decade later is debatable, it was in part a recognition that the NHS could not continue to provide full care and support to meet the demands of individuals with increasingly chronic ill-health. At the same time, evaluation of the impact of EBP from service users' perspectives has been a growing area for research funders such as The National Institute for Health Research (NIHR) in the UK, who are increasingly asking for evidence of collaboration between researchers and users. There is also increased recognition that there has frequently been a mismatch between research that is funded and research that service users would like to see funded (Tallon et al. 2000). A range of initiatives have been established to find common ground in terms of priorities of importance for research from service users' perspectives. One important example is the James Lind Alliance (JLA) which was established to help identify and address uncertainties about the effects of treatment and facilitate the identification of research priorities shared by patients and clinicians (www.lindalliance.org).

In England and Wales, the national advisory group INVOLVE has been instrumental in ensuring users are engaged in all aspects of the research process. In addition other organizations such as the

National Institute for Health and Clinical Excellence (NICE) have paved the way for greater involvement of service users and their carers, ranging from involvement in setting priority topic areas for clinical guideline development, membership of guideline development groups, membership of a Citizens Council to advise NICE decision making, and more recently in strategies to support and sustain the use of NICE guidance in practice. In the UK in 1998, the Healthcare Commission instituted four yearly annual surveys of patient experiences, and in 2001 introduced annual surveys of acute inpatient care. The UK NIHR has been pivotal in ensuring service user representatives are actively engaged as members of research teams contributing to the development, implementation, and evaluation of research commissioned across its funding programs. INVOLVE is funded by the NIHR to support and promote active public involvement in NHS, public health, and social care research (www .invo.org.uk). In England, the NIHR has also funded Collaborations for Leadership in Applied Health Research and Care (CLAHRCS) as a way of implementing research findings into practice, with nine CLAHRCs set up to date across the country. Their main role is to undertake high-quality applied health research focused on the needs of patients and support the translation of research evidence into practice in the NHS. CLAHRCS are collaborative partnerships between a university and its local NHS organizations, focused on improving patient outcomes through the conduct and application of applied health research.

Similar moves to enable those who use the health services to contribute to the development of health service policy, research priorities, and dissemination of findings have been undertaken by bodies tasked with leading national funding priorities in other parts of the world. The Canadian Institutes for Health Research (CIHR) created a conceptual framework for Citizen Engagement which is intended to guide the agency's efforts to meaningfully engage the public in research processes including priority setting. In the USA, service users can receive e-mail updates on a range of work undertaken on behalf of the Agency for Healthcare Research and Quality (AHRQ), including flyers on aspects of health management and work undertaken as part of AHRQs Knowledge Transfer/Implementation Program. The National Health and Medical Research Council of Australia (NHMRC) produces a range of information for service users using media which includes podcasts, guidelines, and health facts on different health priorities. The NHMRC also works with

The Consumers Health Forum of Australia to inform how service users can be included in research.

As much of this work is relatively recent, evidence of the impact of greater involvement of service users in the planning, development, and dissemination of national policy and research priorities is evolving. Staniszewska (2008) highlighted some of the key limitations of this evidence base including differing terminology, poor conceptual or theoretical underpinnings, limited understanding of the concept of impact in this context, and mainly descriptive accounts of impact with little robust measurement. Oliver and colleagues (2004) developed a framework to inform a literature review of how service users were being used in research identification and prioritization in England, identifying data from several sources, including electronic databases and interviews with service users and research program managers. Of 286 documents identified which specifically referred to service users in identifying or prioritizing research topics, most ($n = 91$) were general discussion documents, some of which included a theoretical analysis or a critique of research agendas from a consumer perspective, 160 reported specific efforts to include consumers in identifying or prioritizing research topics, and a further 51 reported consumers identifying or prioritizing research topics in the course of other work. Most of the literature comprised descriptive reports by researchers who were key actors in involving consumers. The authors concluded that if service users are to be engaged, appropriate skills, resources, and time are essential to develop appropriate working practices. The potentially beneficial impact of user involvement in the research process was outlined by Staniszewska et al. (2007) who described the way in which parents influenced the focus of The Parents of Premature Babies Project (POPPY) which undertook research into aspects of neonatal care and provision of services important for the parents of premature babies in terms of aims, methods, ethical aspects, and dissemination. POPPY findings have been submitted to the UK Neonatal Task Force where it is hoped that the model of family-centered care proposed by the study will influence future care provision.

Nevertheless, as Black and Jenkinson (2009) highlight, a number of challenges remain. These include how to engage service users at the outset, what approaches to use to measure service users' experiences and outcomes of care and need to consider methodological issues, practical considerations, and ensure data of interest are the most relevant for the service user. Some of these challenges are addressed later in this chapter.

## The role of service user groups and networks

Input by service users into the work of national agencies in some countries has undoubtedly been influenced by the growth of voluntary and peer advocacy or support groups, established to promote networking among members with the same health problem (e.g., local breast cancer survivor groups), to coordinate lobbying for policy or service change to reflect EBP and user views (e.g., the National Childbirth Trust in the UK) or to coordinate and encourage donations to fund research to improve treatment, patient outcomes, and experiences (e.g., Cancer Research UK). Many groups use the internet to disseminate information, provide links to sources of support and advice and discuss results of latest relevant studies. In some middle-income countries, the importance of user involvement to achieve internationally established targets to improve country-level health is now apparent. For example, in Brazil, women's groups have been actively engaged by national policy makers in work to improve birth outcomes, reduce unnecessary interventions during labor and birth, and highlight where gaps in maternity and infant care practices persist in order to achieve the Millennium Development goals (Diniz et al. 2007). The Health Technology Assessment International Programme has established an international Patient and Public Involvement Group to support those doing research in the field. Further information can be obtained from their web site (www.htai.org).

## Defining EBP priorities and outcomes from a service user perspective

The impact and outcomes of EBP from a service users' perspective needs to reflect a spectrum of involvement from representation on an advisory or service user representation group, to an individual's involvement in decisions about their day-to-day care and management, to or a decision about participation in a research study. The following sections describe impact from a range of perspectives from the macro to the micro-level.

## Engagement in priorities for EBP

Despite the growth in service user support groups, "grass-roots" initiatives and role of national agencies to support user involvement, there was until fairly recently a dearth of information on how user perspectives of the outcomes of EBP could be gauged and utilized to sustain and support change, with little debate or dialogue as to what "research," "evidence," or "impact" mean from the perspective of service users. In the UK there was previously little formal advocacy of how to engage users in research and little reference, if any, in published research reports of how or if service users had been involved (Hanley et al. 2001). Indeed there was no information on the type of involvement or extent of involvement of service users. A UK survey of 62 clinical trials offices and support units on user involvement between 1990 and 1998 found that 23 centers reported that users had already been involved, with most positive about their involvement (Hanley et al. 2001). Of the remaining centers, 17 reported that they had plans to involve service users and 15 had no such plans although only 4 considered their involvement irrelevant. This was the first UK national survey of service user involvement and it highlighted a number of issues including some confusion as to the role users should play and indication that in the main, users contributed to the content of patient information leaflets.

Nearly a decade later there is an extensive and developing evidence base that describes how many different studies have involved service users, for example, INVOLVE maintain a bibliography of relevant studies (www.invo.org.uk) although how to ensure service users are engaged in the identification of research priorities needs further consideration. Stewart and Oliver (2008) conducted a review on behalf of the JLA which considered patients and clinicians research priorities. They developed a framework to identify reported priority setting activities, supported with specialist software. Overall, 258 studies were identified for inclusion, 148 of which reported patients or clinicians engagement with research; 61 of these studies (41.2%) only described broad research areas in terms of populations (5/61), interventions (11/61), outcomes (20/61), or broad research topics (44/61); 96/148 (64.9%) reported patients' or clinicians' identifying research questions; 5/148 (3.4%) reported patients' or clinicians' views on research measures. Clinicians were more likely to be engaged in the identification of clinical research priorities (131/148 studies compared to 27/148) despite policy support for patient and public involvement.

## Engagement in identification of outcomes of EBP

In more recent years there has been growing interest in understanding how knowledge derived from research is disseminated and used in non-academic contexts, with drivers for this change arising from political imperatives, recognition that research-based knowledge has had little impact and need for research funders and advocates to increase rigor in the direction and design of research (Davies & Nutley 2008). Empirical studies of the impact of research which aimed to ascertain how and where the findings of research have been used have tended to focus on positive outcomes for the group targeted by the intervention—for example, a reduction in maternal perineal pain at 10 days as a result of using vicryle rapide suturing material rather than chromic catgut (Kettle et al. 2002). However, what we tend to find is that these outcomes are often imposed from the perspective of the researcher or clinician; they tend to be based on short-term follow-up and rarely take account of the perspectives of the service user. Growing evidence illustrates important discrepancies that exist between health professionals and patients with regards to the way in which a "good outcome" is defined (Hewlett et al. 2005). Outcomes on the whole tend to be quite narrow, do not take account of the consequences for the service user or consider other direct or indirect consequences of the change in practice, including impact on other areas of health-care provision. One example of this was early consensus work to identify important core health domains for the assessment of rheumatoid arthritis which included only clinicians, researchers, members of pharmaceutical companies and economists in the decision-making process (Felson et al. 1993). Pain was identified as a primary outcome. More recently, patients have been involved in this process, and although pain remains an important outcome, fatigue and general well-being are additional outcomes that had not previously been considered (Carr et al. 2003; Hewlett et al. 2005).

The gap between what a "good" clinical outcome means from a health service provider or policy perspective (usually a change in practice which leads to care which is clinically and cost-effective—for further information refer to Chapter 8) and what a "good" outcome means from the perspective of a service user persists. There may also be debate as to why service user views are important, as it is usually the clinician who makes the final decision about the content of care, as Diane Doran refers to in Chapter 4 which describes an outcomes framework. Nevertheless, as Diane also points out, if service user views of outcomes are not collated, clinicians will operate in isolation from knowing if or how their care is effective or resulting in potential harm and greater resource use.

A large UK wide matched pair cluster study (The PEARLS study: www.rcm.org.uk) which aims to improve the assessment and management of perineal trauma following birth included a Delphi study and consensus conference to identify what outcomes women who had sustained perineal trauma considered to be important at different times in their recovery after giving birth. Previous trials of perineal care outcomes, for example, use of different suturing methods and/or suturing materials have tended to use pain as a primary outcome measure, either as a "generic" measure or in relation to a specific activity, for example, resumption of sexual intercourse (Kettle et al. 2002). The PEARLS trial team invited women who had given birth within the previous 6 months at two units not participating in the trial to participate in a social event to take part in a "Who Wants to be a Millionaire" voting process to identify the most important outcomes to them following perineal trauma at 1 week, 2–4 weeks, and 3 months after giving birth. At each event, women were asked to score on a scale of 1–6 using an electronic key pad, how they would rate each of 44 outcomes following perineal trauma by order of importance (1 being not important and 6 being very important).

Of note was that women at both sites did not consider pain outcomes to be the most important issue for them. That their perineal tear or episiotomy did not become infected was women's most important concern at 1 week after the birth. This finding was reflected in the trial as a secondary outcome measure, as lack of routinely collated data on incidence and onset of perineal wound infection meant it could not be used as a primary outcome measure, with sufficient numbers to power the study (see PEARLS protocol, www.rcm.org.uk). Inclusion as a secondary outcome will provide the first evidence of incidence of perineal wound infection within 3 months of birth at a national level which could inform future work. This example illustrates that service users can present a very different perspective on what is important for their health and well-being than that assumed by the researchers, clinicians, and health service providers.

## Patient-reported outcome measures

In addition to the need to consider how service users can be involved in the identification of priority topics and outcomes of EBP, there has been a significant growth in the development and use of instruments more recently referred to as patient-reported outcome measures (PROMs) (Patrick et al. 2007), to assess the impact of implementation on service user outcomes. The following sections outline some of the

PROMS developed and related issues with respect to their use. Some have been developed to assess impact on general health and well-being, whereas others have been developed to assess a particular condition or procedure (Garratt et al. 2002). Of note is that collation of evidence of service user outcomes tends to be purported to be used as feedback to clinicians and service providers (e.g., through audit) with the expectation that it will improve *future* health outcomes and quality of care—the extent to which findings are used to improve the *current* health and well-being of the individual respondent is less clear.

## Service user reported outcomes of care

When assessing the impact of an intervention to implement EBP, the researcher or clinician can make a number of subjective or objective assessments of "benefit." However, it is the individual who has been the recipient of the intervention who can provide a unique insight with respect to the impact of an intervention on their own physical or emotional well-being, their quality of life, and experiences. The issue for use of EBP is how this evidence is used and how to ensure the service user's perceptions of what is important to them is captured as highlighted earlier.

Growing interest in capturing the patient perspective of ill-health and the relative impact of health care has resulted in the development of several hundred instruments that purport to capture the patient perspective (Garratt 2009; Garratt et al. 2002). Variably referred to as measures of quality of life, health-related quality of life, or health status, more recent guidance adopts the term *Patient-reported Outcome Measures* (PROMs) (Patrick et al. 2007). Well-developed PROMs, usually self-completed questionnaires, aim to provide a systematic and structured assessment of the patient's perspective across a range of health concerns, from symptoms and physical functioning to well-being and quality of life (Fitzpatrick et al. 1998).

There are two broad categories of PROM: generic and specific. Generic measures are not age-, disease-, or treatment-specific and contain multiple concepts of health-related quality of life relevant to both patients and the general public, supporting their application in both population groups (Garratt et al. 2002). Population-based normal values can be calculated which supports data interpretation.

There are two classes of generic measure: health profiles and utility measures. Examples of widely used generic health profile and utility measures are the Short Form 36-item Health Survey (SF-36, Ware & Sherbourne 1992) and the EuroQoL EQ-5D (EuroQoL Group 1990; www.euroqol.org) respectively.

Historically, PROMs have been used in clinical trials and research settings. However, growing interest in capturing the patient's perspective in a routine practice has been fueled by suggestions that the value of health care remains unclear until its impact and effectiveness is assessed using outcomes relevant to patients and health professionals (Department of Health 2008a). This led to the recent implementation of specific PROMs within the NHS. From 2009, the Department of Health in England has required all providers of elective surgery for NHS patients to use PROMs data to assess the outcomes of four commonly performed elective procedures: hip replacement, knee replacement, groin hernia repair, and varicose vein surgery. The EuroQoL EQ-5D is the recommended generic measure, to be used alongside specific measures for each condition: the Oxford Hip Score (Dawson et al. 1996), the Oxford Knee Score, and the Aberdeen Varicose Vein Questionnaire;

Improvement in clinical quality and outcome is at the heart of current NHS reforms in England:

> *"Effectiveness of care. This means understanding success rates from different treatments for different conditions. Assessing this will include clinical measures such as mortality or survival rates and measures of clinical improvement. Just as important is the effectiveness of care from the patient's own perspective which will be measured through patient-reported outcomes measures (PROMs)…"*
>
> *High Quality Care for All: NHS Next Stage Review (Department of Health, 2008a)*

It is envisaged that PROMs data will be used by service commissioners, clinicians, managers, and regulators to benchmark provider care across the NHS and by service users to evaluate the relative clinical quality of services, hence acting to benchmark provider care across the NHS (Department of Health 2008b). Moreover, the data will inform the appropriateness of referrals, while providing evidence of service efficacy and cost-effectiveness. Service users may use the information to inform their choice of health-care provider. Data will be aggregated and analysed prior to being presented as standard reports to the Department of Health.

Bream and Black (2009) undertook a systematic search of studies to identify those in which patient and clinician reports of health status and complications of the four elective surgical procedures selected for use of PROMs in the NHS were reported. Of 62 studies identified, 23 were for hip and 33 for knee disease, with few studies of outcomes following the other procedures. Studies of post-operative complications were more limited with only 12 studies reporting on surgical site infection and one on urinary tract infection. No studies were reported on lower respiratory tract infections. Despite wide variations in findings, there were patterns which in the main related to outcomes of undergoing arthroplasty. Patient and clinician views of health status had moderate correlation when both were reporting on the same dimension of health status with respect to disability. The researchers found huge variation with how post-operative complications were measured. Nevertheless, they concluded that clinicians, service providers, commissioners, and policy makers could be confident that patients' reports could provide an accurate assessment of the outcome of elective surgery.

As described above, several domains can be included in PROMs as long as they are specific to the clinical area of interest. The availability of sites such as the Patient-Reported Outcome and Quality of Life database (www.proqoild.org) which lists over 600 instruments (accessed 08/07/2009) may be useful when deciding which one(s) to use, although not all of those listed may have data on their validity, reliability, and feasibility, important issues to consider when deciding if an instrument is appropriate for the intended target population. For example, in the UK there is increasing concern that more women are developing pressure ulcers during labor. Pressure ulcers appear to be more likely to occur in women who have a high BMI or conversely in women with a low BMI, possibly due to lack of mobilization during labor or the friction of monitoring equipment placed on the woman's abdomen during labor. As a consequence, some maternity units are including the Waterlow Pressure Ulcer Risk Assessment score (Waterlow 1985) in their routine maternity records to be used to assess all women in their care. Although this is not an instrument to be completed by the service user, it illustrates the need to consider the appropriateness of an outcome measure. The Waterlow score has not been validated for women during pregnancy, the age ranges included on the risk score are not relevant for women of child-bearing age; it includes a male/female gender category and there is no evidence of the optimal time to use the measure on a woman in pregnancy. This highlights the issue of need to develop population-specific instruments or at least validate instruments and measures for specific populations.

The extent to which outcome measures collated in the PROMs, which include domains of function, disability, and aspects of quality of life, relate to service user views of outcomes important to them as opposed to clinician and health service provider and funder interest is debatable. There are also limitations with respect to the validity and generalizability of PROMs for different population groups and different clinical symptoms. There is also a lack of information on complications the service user may have experienced which may not be collated on a PROM.

Fitzpatrick and colleagues (1998) undertook a review funded by the NHS Health Technology Assessment programme to evaluate patient-based outcome measures for use in clinical trials. They identified that concepts, definitions, and theories to inform how or why the measure was developed were not clearly or consistently used. They recommended that eight questions should be considered by researchers when deciding which outcome measures to use.

- Is the content of the instrument appropriate to the questions which the clinical trial is intended to address? (Appropriateness)
- Does the instrument produce results that are reproducible and internally consistent? (Reliability)
- Does the instrument measure what it claims to measure? (Validity)
- Does the instrument detect changes over time that matter to patients? (Responsiveness)
- How precise are the scores of the instrument? (Precision)
- How interpretable are the scores of the instrument? (Interpretability)
- Is the instrument acceptable to patients? (Acceptability)
- Is the instrument easy to administer and process? (Feasibility)

Box 7.1 includes examples of some of the more commonly used PROMS to assess service user outcomes, including generic instruments

**Box 7.1  Examples of PROMS to assess service user outcomes of care**

| Instrument/Measure | Dimensions |
|---|---|
| *Generic* | |
| Short-Form 36 (SF36) (Ware & Sherbourne 1992) | Eight domains related to aspects of physical and psychological health, disability |
| EQ-5D (EuroQual Europe Group 1990) | Health related quality of life, including health status; utility. Provides a single index value for health status |
| *Psychological* | |
| Edinburgh Postnatal Depression Scale (EPDS) (Cox et al. 1987) | Aspects of psychological well-being during previous 7 days |
| Beck Depression Inventory (BDI (Beck 1961), BDI I-A, BDI-II (Beck et al. 1996) | Multiple-choice self-report inventory to measure the severity of depression |
| *Condition specific* | |
| Oxford Hip Score (Dawson et al. 1996) | Impairment, symptoms, disability |
| Minessota living with heart failure questionnaire (Rector et al. 1993) | Specific quality of life measure for individuals with congestive heart failure to assess perceptions of the effects of heart failure and its treatment on their daily life |
| Migraine Specific Quality of Life (MSQOL, Santenello et al. 1995) | To assess needs-based quality of life across 5 domains within 24hrs of a migraine attack |
| Seattle Angina Questionnaire (SAQ) (Spertus et al. 1995) | To quantify the physical and emotional effects of coronary artery disease over previous 4 weeks |
| *Pain* | |
| Short-form McGill Pain Questionnaire (SF-MPQ-2) (Melzack 1987) | Measure of pain symptoms of both neuropathic and non-neuropathic pain conditions during previous 7 days |

which could inform comparison of outcomes across different health conditions, instruments developed to assess physical or psychological health and well-being, and site-specific outcomes. Some instruments also provide a measure of utility (utility measures have been developed from economics and decision theory to provide an estimate of individual service users' overall preferences for different health states) (Drummond et al. 1993).

Heterogeneity between instruments and measures and use across different acute and chronic health conditions may limit the extent to which service user outcomes can be compared. There is also an important need to develop instruments which measure service user reported complications as a consequence of the original intervention (e.g., needing additional treatment from primary care sources for a surgical site infection following discharge home, which the acute care sector is not collating as an outcome) if we are to really understand outcomes beyond initial implementation. From the perspective of EBP, we also have to ensure that if measures informed by evidence of outcomes important to service users are developed, findings are accorded equal priority with other forms of evidence.

## Service user reported experiences of care

> "If quality is to be at the heart of everything we do, it must be understood from the perspective of patients."
>
> *High Quality Care for All: NHS Next Stage Review (Department of Health, 2008a)*

In addition to work to identify service users' views on the outcomes of their care, researchers have also become interested in measuring users' *experiences* of the humanity and dignity of their care, outcomes of which can also improve quality of care. Surveys of service user experiences can also gauge trends and patterns to see how common certain experiences are. The Picker Institute Europe is a research charity and advocate for patient-centered health care. Based on their work with service users, surveys developed by the Picker Institute to measure experiences of health care cover eight quality dimensions (Picker Institute Europe 2009) highlighted by service users as of importance to them:

- fast access to reliable health advice
- effective treatment delivered by trusted professionals
- participation in decisions and respect for preferences
- clear, comprehensible information and support for self-care
- attention to physical and environmental needs
- emotional support, empathy, and respect
- involvement of, and support for, family and carers
- continuity of care and smooth transitions

A tool kit produced by the Picker Institute aims to support health-care staff to collect data on service user experiences and how to use data to enhance quality of health-care provision (Picker Institute Europe 2009). They recommend that surveys of service users should include specific factual questions about what happened to them during their health-care journey. Examples of questions include "reporting" style questions such as:

*Q: Did a member of staff tell you about medication side effects to watch for when you went home?* (Picker Institute Europe 2009: p. 2)

Black and Jenkinson (2009) cite questions included in Picker Institute questionnaires for the evaluation of inpatient care as good examples of well-designed instruments (Box 7.2).

Topics covered and phrasing of questions were derived from preliminary qualitative inquiries, which included in-depth interviews with patients and pilot testing of draft questionnaires (Black & Jenkinson 2009). These examples provide useful information as

---

**Box 7.2 Examples of questions to elicit service user experiences of care**

*Q: When you had important questions to ask the doctor, did you get answers you could understand?*
*Response options: Yes, always; Yes, sometimes; No; I had not need to ask*
*Q: Were you involved as much as you wanted to be in decisions about your care and treatment?*
*Response options: Yes, definitely; Yes, to some extent; No*
Picker Institute: cited Black and Jenkinson (2009)

they highlight precisely where the problems are and what could be done to improve the particular elements of care for the service user. Narrative accounts may have a limited value in audits of routine care but can provide rich insights useful for service providers, users, and their carers.

Service users' perspectives of outcomes with implications for their health, well-being, and experiences of care are not the only issue of interest following use of EBP. A growing area of concern for UK and other health providers and policy makers internationally is the safety and quality of care, with the number of adverse or near-miss events rising (Leape et al. 2002), including those recorded in maternity care (Smith & Dixon 2007). Women's views of safety are important as they are the ones who will suffer if things go wrong. As their behavior is part of the process of unsafe practice, as such they are also part of the solution. A team from the Picker Institute recently completed a qualitative study of women's views of the safety of their maternity care, findings from which informed an inquiry into the maternity services in England undertaken by The King's Fund, an independent charitable foundation (Magee & Askham 2008). Women who had recently given birth were asked a number of questions relating to their understanding of risk in childbirth; what safe and unsafe care in childbirth meant to them; what contributory factors related to safety did they have concerns about with respect to their own birth experience; and if they had had a previous birth, if they considered their most recent experience was as safe or was less safe. One to one interviews were conducted with 31 women purposively selected to represent a range of age, ethnicity, parity and place, and mode of birth.

Women's views highlighted a number of important issues. "Unsafe" care included perceptions of lack of staff, being left alone in labor, poor monitoring, and not knowing who was caring for them. Giving birth in hospital was perceived by some women to reduce the risk of something going wrong, whereas others mentioned home as a better place to birth and that the local hospital itself could be a risk factor. Safety did not appear to be a major preoccupation of the women interviewed; if women felt unsafe it was because they did not know what to expect or because they had been concerned over staffing levels. What was clear from the interviews was that the bond and the trust a woman formed with the midwife providing her care was influential in a woman achieving what she viewed as a positive outcome. As the researchers highlight the nature of birth means that awareness of safety factors often listed as significant in influencing outcomes can be affected during labor itself by pain or pain relief and ultimately by the delivery of a healthy baby (Magee & Askham 2008).

The growth of internet technology has also resulted in innovations with respect to how service users can share their experiences and outcomes of health care with others and with respect to the application and completion of PROMS. Healthtalk Online' is a web site which enables those who access the site to hear about others experiences of health and illness through videoed interviews (www.healthtalkonline.org). The information posted on the web site is based on qualitative research into patient experiences led by researchers from the University of Oxford. A range of conditions are addressed; cancer, mental health, living with dying, pregnancy and childbirth, bones and joints, heart disease, living with disability, and chronic health issues. Under each heading are a range of subject-related topics which the visitor to the web site can click onto to hear an individual's account of the impact of news of a condition on them, the effects on their relationships, work and social life, decisions about treatment, and side effects of treatment.

Some very sensitive areas are addressed, for example, how to cope with the loss of a loved one and the practical aspects which have to be considered such as arranging a funeral. As these issues are presented from the perspective of the person who has suffered the condition or the loss, they are very powerful stories. The research team have recently launched another area of the web site which enables service users who have participated in clinical trials to relate their experiences, including why they did or did not wish to participate as well as practical issues of what taking part in a clinical trial actually meant from their perspective.

## Addressing the challenges and developing the evidence base

### The challenges

As referred to earlier in this chapter, evidence of what outcomes service users consider to be important is evolving but many challenges remain if their views are not to be perceived as an "add on" to strategies to enhance use of EBP. Clearer concepts and definitions of service user outcomes in health service organization, evaluation, and development are also required, as is work to develop the most appropriate "metrics" to capture the impact of service user involvement (Staniszewska et al. 2008).

Challenges include working with service users to identify which outcomes they determine as important, to develop and validate the most robust measures of these and ensure sample sizes to inform comparisons are adequate to detect differences which are statistically meaningful (Black & Jenkinson 2009). If we want outcome measures to be meaningful for service users, we also need more work into understanding the relationship between a person's experiences and their reported health outcomes—for example, will a poor experience of care (e.g., a dirty ward, poor food or reporting that staff were rude) influence a person's views of other outcomes including impact on their health.

It is also important that researchers can take any potential bias into account, for example people with a debilitating illness may be less likely to respond to an outcome survey than those who are healthy. When to question a service user about their views of an outcome is also an important area for consideration. There has been debate in the maternity services that if surveys of care are undertaken very soon after the birth, findings may well be influenced by the "halo" effect of a woman and her partner being overjoyed at the safe birth of their child, feelings which may well dissipate if a longer length of time after the birth was selected to measure their views of outcomes. Similarly, if the length of time between the "event" and the outcome of interest is too long, there is the risk of introducing recall bias. Given that many of us work in health areas caring for people from many different ethnic groups, we need further work to determine how those from different cultures view a positive outcome of care.

There are some positive moves in some areas of the UK NHS to ensure data on service users outcomes and experiences are used to inform practice, although at the moment these appear to be driven by financial incentives rather than the service user perspectives per se (Black & Jenkinson 2009). From a political and policy agenda, service user involvement is key to achieving and sustaining safe, high-quality care (Department of Health 2008a); the challenge is to ensure their involvement remains a key priority as they can be a source of change as the episiotomy example from the UK demonstrates.

## Developing the evidence base

As Staniszewska and colleagues (2008) highlight, the international research base to underpin service user involvement is partial and lacks coherence. Currently those wishing to engage service users in views of their outcomes have to rely on previously developed measures which may not have been evaluated for that particular group of people or the setting within which care was received. We have examples in other chapters of this book of how use of EBP has been defined and captured from multiple perspectives, although evidence of service user engagement is frequently missing. If we are to develop a robust evidence base, several issues have to be considered. Researchers considering use of models or frameworks to support research use in practice need to consider how user involvement could be reflected and if current models/frameworks would need to be adapted to achieve this. We also require evidence of indirect or longer-term impacts of evidence use which could influence outcomes (positively or negatively) for the service user. Reliance on self-report measures and surveys of service users may not be sufficient to understand more fully the complexity of outcomes of EBP on health-care organizations, care systems, and processes across the primary and secondary care sectors which ultimately impact on the individuals receiving our care.

## Acknowledgments

We would like to thank Dr Sophie Staniszewska and Dr Kirstie Haywood of Warwick University for their comments on the original draft of this chapter.

## References

Beck, A.T. (1961). *Depression: Causes and Treatment*. Philadelphia: University of Pennsylvania.

Beck, A.T., Steer, R.A., Ball, R., & Ranieri, W. (1996). Comparison of Beck Depression Inventories-IA and -II in psychiatric outpatients. *Journal of Personality Assessment*, 67(3), 588–597.

Black, N. & Jenkinson, C. (2009). Measuring patient's experiences and outcomes. *British Medical Journal*, 339, 2495.

Bream, E. & Black, N. (2009). What is the relationship between patients' and clinicians' reports of the outcomes of elective surgery? *Journal Health Service Research Policy*, 14(3), 174–182.

Carr, A., Hewlett, S., Hughes, R. et al. (2003). Rheumatology outcomes: The patient's perspective. *Journal of Rheumatology*, 30, 880–883.

Carroli, G. & Mignini, L. (2008). Episiotomy for vaginal birth. *Cochrane Database of Systematic Reviews*, 3, CD000081. DOI: 10.1002/14651858. CD000081.pub2

Cox, J.L., Holden, J.M., & Sagovsky, R. (1987). Detection of postnatal depression. Development of the 10-item Edinburgh Postnatal Depression Scale. *British Journal of Psychiatry*, 150, 782–786.

Davies, H. & Nutley, S. (2008). Learning more about how research-based knowledge gets used: Guidance in the development of new empirical research—Working paper. William T. Grant Foundation. Available online: www.wtgrantfoundation.org.

Dawson, J., Fitzpatrick, R., Carr, A., & Murray, D. (1996). Questionnaire on the perceptions of patients about total hip replacement. *The Journal of Bone and Joint Surgery: British Volume*, 78(2), 185–190.

Department of Health (1999). *Saving Lives: Our Healthier Nation*. London: Crown.

Department of Health (2008a). *High Quality Care for All—NHS Next Stage Review Final Report*. London: The Stationery Office.

Department of Health (2008b). *The NHS in England: The Operating Framework for 2008/09*. London: The Stationery Office.

Drummond, M., Torrance, G., & Mason, J. (1993). Cost-effectiveness league tables: More harm than good? Social Science & Medicine, 37(1), 33–40.

Diniz, S., Bick, D., Bastos, M.H., & Riesco, M. (2007). Empowering women in Brazil. *The Lancet*, 370, 1596–1598.

EuroQoL Group (1990). EuroQol—A new facility for the measurement of health-related quality of life. *Health Policy*, 16, 199–208.

Felson, D.T., Anderson, J.J., Boers, M. et al. (1993). The American College of Rheumatology preliminary core set of disease activity measures for rheumatoid arthritis clinical trials. The Committee on Outcome Measures in Rheumatoid Arthritis Clinical Trials. *Arthritis and Rheumatism*, 36(6), 729–740.

Fitzpatrick, R., Davy, C., Buxton, M.J., & Jones, D.R. (1998). Evaluating patient-based outcome measures for use in clinical trials. *Health Technology Assessment*, 2(14), 1–4.

Garratt, A.M. (2009). Editorial. Patient reported outcome measures in trials. *British Medical Journal*, 338, a2597.

Garratt, A.M., Schmidt, L., Mackintosh, A., & Fitzpatrick, R. (2002). Quality of life measurement: Bibliographic study of patient assessed health outcome measures. *British Medical Journal*, 324, 1417–1419.

Graham, I.D. (1996). I believe therefore I practise. *The Lancet*, 347, 4–5.

Graham, I.D., Carroli, G., Davies, C., & Medves, J.M. (2005). Episiotomy rates around the world: An update. *Birth*, 32(3), 219–223.

Graham, I.D., Logan, J., Harrison, M.B. et al. (2006). Lost in knowledge translation: Time for a map? *Journal of Continuing Education of the Health Professions*, 26(13), 13–24.

Hanley, B., Truesdale, A., King, A., Elbourne, D., & Chalmers, I. (2001). Involving consumers in designing, conducting, and interpreting randomised controlled trials: Questionnaire survey. *British Medical Journal*, 322, 519–523.

Hewlett, S., Kirwan. J., Pollock, J. et al. (2005). Patient initiated outpatient follow up in rheumatoid arthritis: Six year randomised controlled trial. *British Medical Journal*, 330(7484), 171.

Kettle, C., Hills, R.K., Jones, P., Darby, L., Gray, R., & Johanson, R. (2002). Continuous versus interrupted perineal repair with standard or rapidly absorbed sutures after spontaneous vaginal birth: A randomised controlled trial. *The Lancet*, 359, 2217–2223.

Leape, L., Berwick, D., & Bates, D. (2002). What practices will most improve safety? Evidence-based medicine meets patient safety. *JAMA: The Journal of the American Medical Association*, 288(4), 501–507.

Magee, H. & Askham, J. (2008). Women's views about safety in maternity care. A qualitative study. London: King's Fund.

McGlynn, E., Asch, S.M., Adams, J. et al. (2003). The quality of health care delivered to adults in the United States. *New England Journal of Medicine*, 348, 2635–2645.

Melzack, R. (1987). The short-form McGill Pain Questionnaire. *Pain*, 30(2), 191–197.

Oliver, S., Clarke-Jones, L., Rees, R., et al. (2004). Involving consumers in research and development agenda setting for the NHS: developing an evidence-based approach. *Health Technology Assessment*, 8(15), 1–148.

Patrick, D.L., Burke, L.B., Powers, J.H. et al. (2007). Patient-reported outcomes to support medical product labeling claims: FDA perspective. *Value Health*, 10(Suppl. 2), S125–S137.

Picker Institute Europe (2009). Using patient feedback. Downloaded from www.pickereurope.org (last accessed July 27, 2009).

Rector, T.S., Kubo, S.H., & Cohn, J.N. (1993). Validity of the Minnesota Living With Heart Failure Questionnaire as a Measure of Therapeutic Response to Enalapril or Placebo. *American Journal of Cardiology*, 71, 1106–1107.

Santanello, N.C., Hartmaier, S.L., Epstein, R.S., & Silberstein, S.D. (1995). Validation of a new quality of life questionnaire for acute migraine headache. *Headache*, 35(6), 330–337.

Schuster, M., McGlynn, E., & Brook, R.H. (1998). How good is the quality of health care in the United States? *Milbank Quarterly*, 76, 517–563.

Smith, A. & Dixon, A. (2007). *The Safety of Maternity Services in England*. London: King's Fund.

Spertus, J.A., Winder, J.A., Dewhurst, T.A. et al. (1995). Development and evaluation of the Seattle Angina Questionnaire: A new functional status measure for coronary artery disease. *Journal of the American College of Cardiology*, 25(2), 333–341.

Staniszewska, S., Jones, N., Newburn, M., & Marshall, S. (2007). User involvement in the development of a research bid: Barriers, enablers and impacts. *Health Expectations*, 10, 173–183.

Staniszewska, S. (2008). Measuring the impact of patient and public involvement: the need for an evidence base. *International Journal for Quality in Health Care*, 20(6), 373–374.

Staniszewska, S., Herron-Marx, S., & Mockford, C. (2008). Measuring the impact of patient and public involvement: The need for an evidence base—Editorial. *International Journal for Quality in Health Care*, 20(6), 373–374.

Stewart, R. & Oliver, S. (2008). A systematic map of studies of patients' and clinicians' research priorities. London: James Lind Alliance.

Tallon, D., Chard, J., & Dieppe, P. (2000). Relation between agendas of the research community and the research consumer. *The Lancet*, 355, 2037–2040.

Tarpey, M. (2006). Why people get involved in health and social care research. INVOLVE Support Unit. Available online: www.invo.org.uk.

Ware, J. & Sherbourne, C. (1992). The MOS 36-item shortform health survey (SF-36). I. Conceptual framework and item selection. *Medical Care*, 30, 473–483.

Waterlow, J. (1985). Pressure sores: A risk assessment card. *Nursing Times*, 81(48), 49–55.

# Chapter 8

# Evaluating the impact of implementation on economic outcomes

*Lisa Gold*

---

**Key learning points**

- The economic impact of a change in practice is the value of outcomes, relative to the investment required.
- Economic evaluation provides a well-developed framework to weigh up the costs and consequences for different groups that arise from any change in practice.
- Assessing economic impact requires measurement of resources invested in practice change, as well as outcomes that result.
- Evaluation of evidence-based practice needs to always include economic impact, to ensure practice change really does create more good than harm.

---

## Introduction

Most evaluations of evidence-based practice (EBP) do not consider the impact on economic outcomes. Some argue that financial cost should have no role in health sector decision making, that consideration of such impact is even unethical (Williams 1998) and there is ongoing debate that the impact on economic outcomes can and should be assessed only after a statistically and clinically significant impact on outcomes has been demonstrated. In this chapter I will argue that evaluations of EBP should always consider the impact on economic outcomes, that it is unethical *not* to do so, and that while a two-stage process is possible in theory, it is rarely achieved in practice. To do this, we first need a common understanding of what economic outcomes are and of why economists are interested in these outcomes. Then we will look at how these economic outcomes can be assessed in evaluation of EBP. Finally, I will argue that this economic evaluation is an essential part of any evaluation of EBP, that it is the ethical way to proceed, and that it needs to be part of a single approach to evaluation.

# Economics

## What are economic outcomes?

To most people, economics is another word for costs, so it follows that "economic outcomes" of a change in practice is another term for financial cost. To an economist however, economic outcomes of a change in practice are the benefits of that change in practice, in terms of the value attached to all of the consequences that result from that change, for all stakeholders. However, as any change in practice is the result of a choice that has been made to implement change, there is always an "opportunity cost" in terms of the possibility that changing practice has led to an increase in the inputs required for practice, compared to what happened before the change. Inputs such as staff time, equipment, office space, etc. always have some alternative use, in which they would generate benefits of value to the same or another group of people. Therefore, any change in practice which increases use of these resources has an associated opportunity cost, in terms of the lost opportunity to use these resources elsewhere.

Economists therefore cannot let themselves consider the joy of the benefits of implemented practice change without weighing these against the possible harms that result from an increase in economic costs (the financial representation of all resources invested in the practice). To make things more confusing, economic costs are different to accounting costs, as economists will want to include all resources invested in the practice, regardless of whether or not these resources actually have to be paid for (e.g., patients' time). This act of weighing up the benefits that result from a change in practice against the additional costs of that change is called economic evaluation.

## Economics jargon and where economists are coming from

As illustrated in the above section on costs and outcomes, economists working in health care (or education, environment, transport, etc.) suffer from a tendency to speak in a language only vaguely related to English. The result is a set of terms that have one meaning in lay language and another, often critically different, meaning in economics. There are now glossaries available that can be a useful translation tool when dealing with economists (Shiell et al. 2002).

Economics is a social science and is essentially the study of how people make choices when they interact with one another in society. Most of the choices involve giving up something the person has (for most of us, hours of our own time) in order to receive something else (for most of us, money in the form of a wage). We do not do this to get money, but rather to get the things that we can exchange that money for, such as housing, food, clothes, travel, holidays, and so on. Why do we do this? To an economist, human behavior is driven by the search for happiness, or "utility" in economics jargon. Economists differ on what exactly can count as utility, but in general the discipline assumes that people make choices to maximize the utility (happiness) that accrues to the individual (or the household) over a lifetime. The discipline of economics is then based on dual aspects of these choices: the *efficiency* with which such choices are made (do choices maximize utility?); and the *equity* of the distribution of resources people start with and/or of the goods and services people end up with (who has what to start with and who ends up with what?).

It is important to note here that money is not a thing of value in and of itself; it is only a means of trading what we have for what we want. The same concept applies in evaluation: money is not an outcome in itself; it is just a handy way of expressing the value of resources invested in a practice.

### Efficiency, inefficiencies and the case for government intervention

In a perfect world, people would make choices that, with some degree of random error, did mean that they maximized their utility given the resources they had available. The implication would be that any attempt to interfere or intervene in people's exchanges (their trading of what they have for what they want) would lead to suboptimal outcomes in terms of the utility of all people.

However, perfect worlds are useful for theoretical models but do not usually exist in reality. In the real world, departures from the perfect world ideal happen all the time. Take the example of buying lunch at work. The perfect world assumes that I know all the alternatives available to me and all the relevant attributes (or characteristics) of all these alternatives. That means I know all of the different foods that I could purchase, the opening times and location of each shop, and the extent to which each of the foods would satisfy my desires for hunger–satiation, nutrition, taste, texture, etc. The perfect world also assumes that all of the food alternatives have a price that reflects only the investment of land, labor, and capital (equipment) needed to produce them, nothing more. If some of the alternatives (or their ingredients) have been affected by government subsidies, their price will be artificially low and my choice could become biased from the efficient ideal. Conversely, any food shop that can keep out competition may be able to charge artificially high prices and similarly bias my choice. My own perceptions of available alternatives and of what impact they will each have on my desired outcomes (hunger–satiation, nutrition, etc.) could be biased by advertising or by my own lack of information-processing skills due to insufficient education (in turn, the impact of my prior choices and of the inequality of the distribution of initial resources, i.e., where, when, and to whom I was born).

If the choice of lunch now seems exceedingly complicated, turn now to the choice of what interventions to provide in health care. Individuals are rarely fully informed of the alternatives available to address a health-care need and of what outcomes each of these alternatives is likely to have. Indeed, individuals are often unaware of the details of their own health-care need, or even that they have a need that can be addressed by a health-care intervention. In health-care choices, individuals are often represented by a health-care professional (nurse, midwife, family doctor, etc.) who acts as their agent and helps the individual to make an efficient decision. But agents are human too and are themselves subject to a range of incentives (costs and benefits to them resulting from different choices) that may bias their actions away from those most likely to maximize utility of the patient.

In short, it is widely accepted that there are many sectors of a country's economy (or structure) where government can intervene to improve the outcomes for the population compared to what would happen if everyone were left to make their own decisions. Sometimes this is based on equity concerns, but largely this argument is based on efficiency concerns, that government intervention in the funding and/or provision of services can increase the utility of the people compared to the decisions that would be made without government intervention. The extent and format of government intervention varies across different countries, but usually covers at least part of the sectors relating to health care, education, community services, public transport, environment, and defence.

However, government intervention means that we need to find an alternative way to assess whether a proposed change in practice is a good or a bad idea. If government intervention is justified by the lack of knowledge of individuals about the potential relative benefits and harms of different treatment options (often a major reason in health care), then we cannot use individuals' choices to evaluate those treatment options. If government intervention, on equity or efficiency grounds, results in individuals facing subsidized or zero costs for treatment (as for many health-care services), again we cannot use individual choice to evaluate the relative value of different treatment options, because those individuals are no longer weighing up the relative benefits of different options against their (full) relative costs. We need to move the decision to a level higher-up the decision-making structure. This is what happens in health care; we make a decision whether or not to implement change for the whole hospital (or the whole health-care system) and then that decision applies to all of the individuals treated.

Economic evaluation in health care is therefore not the individual sort of economic evaluation that we all make subconsciously every day when we buy lunch or make any other purchasing and investment decisions. The type of economic evaluation that health economists are involved in concerns groups of people, not individuals, and therefore we are looking at the benefits that are created for a group of people due to a change in practice and the change in resource use required in making that change in practice for that group. As we are looking at groups and not individuals, economic evaluation in health care needs to know the average outcome (benefit) and the average resource use (cost) and it is these average estimates that will influence decision making.

It will always be the case that some individuals within the group may experience greater benefits and lower costs than others. This means that a decision made on the basis of the group average may not be the same decision that would be made on an individual level for every individual in that group. This is one of the downsides of group-level decision making. It can always be assessed if the evidence we have can be reliably broken down to a subgroup or individual level, as we could then assess whether a practice change that is judged to be not worthwhile for the whole group may still be worthwhile for a smaller subset. Even then, however, we would need to ensure that any such subset could be reliably identified and somehow separated from the full group if we were to feasibly implement practice change for only a subset of the whole group.

## Equity and the missing side of economics

Economic evaluation is essentially a study of efficiency (getting the maximum utility, or happiness, from the resources that we have available). In practice, while the discipline of economics has dual concerns of efficiency and equity, the practice of economic evaluation is concerned overwhelmingly with efficiency. Equity concerns (analyzing who pays for health care, who accesses health care and/or who gains the benefits of health care) are either completely missing-in-action, or are parked at the door and only sometimes addressed as an afterthought. There are areas of health economics that look at equity in detail (e.g., in trying to improve formulae for the allocation of budgets to match clinical need), but these are separate to the practice of economic evaluation. However, a well-trained economist will always be aware of their missing half, and there are attempts underway to bring some consideration of equity back into the practice of economic evaluation (Cookson et al. 2009).

## Economic evaluation of EBP

Economic evaluation is a large part of what health economists do and there are many textbooks available that set out what economic evaluation is and how to do it. For many, the bible is Methods for the Economic Evaluation of Health Care Programmes by Drummond and colleagues, currently in its third edition (Drummond et al. 2005). A more detailed coverage of issues in economic evaluation is provided in the summary of the United States Panel on Cost-Effectiveness in Health and Medicine (Gold et al. 1996); there are also more straightforward or simplified guides to economic evaluation in health care available (Jefferson et al. 2000). This section simply touches on the wealth of detail covered in these textbooks and any reader interested in how to actually do an economic evaluation should go straight out and buy a copy of the Drummond book.

## Evaluation and economic evaluation

Economic evaluation is part of the evaluation process. By definition, an economic evaluation is a comparative assessment of one practice against another (i.e., an evaluation). The thing that makes it an economic evaluation is that it looks at both the consequences (outcomes) of the alternatives being evaluated and the costs of each alternative (the resources that need to be invested to deliver each alternative, plus the impact of each alternative on future resource use).

## Forms of economic evaluation and more jargon

Economic evaluation can take many forms, with terms such as cost-effectiveness, cost-utility, and cost-benefit widely used (often incorrectly) to describe economic evaluation. Ultimately, there are two forms of economic evaluation: one that can tell you whether the consequences are worth the costs and one that cannot. The former is cost-benefit analysis (CBA) and requires some process to put a monetary valuation on the incremental outcomes of a change in practice (see below). The latter is generally termed cost-effectiveness analysis; this is by far the most common form of economic evaluation in health care and includes economic evaluations of the form of cost-consequences analysis, cost-effectiveness analysis, and cost-utility analysis. Cost-effectiveness analysis does not mean that decisions cannot be made on the worth of EBP change, it simply means that the results of the economic evaluation set out what are the additional costs and additional outcomes of a change in practice, and this information then needs to be presented to a third party (politician, manager, some form of "decision maker") who will judge whether the additional outcomes are worth the additional costs.

## Three steps of economic evaluation

Regardless of the form chosen, there are essentially three steps to economic evaluation:

(1) Identify all of the costs and consequences that are relevant to the practice being evaluated;
(2) Measure all of the items identified; and
(3) Value all of the measured items.

This may seem like an incredibly simple recipe for an activity that in practice can add 10% or more to an evaluation budget, but the core concepts really are this simple. The problems arise when we try to apply these core concepts in practice.

The first problems arise in identification, as we cannot identify relevant costs and consequences until we can (a) define exactly what the practice change under evaluation is, (b) specify the perspective of the evaluation, and (c) state whether we are interested in only the relative performance of the alternatives or also in their absolute impact. In this chapter we will assume that the practice change under evaluation has already been clarified to the extent that it can be clearly described, in terms of who does what to whom, when, and with what intentions. Identification therefore has to first address questions of evaluation perspective and of evaluation context.

### The importance of perspective in evaluation

Economists often come into conflict with the rest of the evaluation team when it comes to the question of perspective in evaluation design. Perspective refers to the point of view taken in the analysis in terms of which costs and consequences are considered as relevant. The perspective follows from the research question as it is determined by the question: "Whose point of view is the evaluation designed to address?" The conflict perhaps arises because the importance of perspective is more obvious in the consideration of costs than in the consideration of consequences. A change in practice can be efficient (or cost-effective) from the point of view of the hospital if it results in reduced costs to the hospital and outcomes for hospital staff and patients that either remain the same or are improved. However, this same practice change could be associated with increased costs for other government services (e.g., general practice, social services, education) and/or for patients' families and it could be associated with increased carer burden, reducing health, and welfare outcomes for carers. Therefore a change that is a good idea from the hospital's perspective may not be such a good idea from the perspective of whole-of-government or of society overall.

A recent example from Australian community child health illustrates a common problem in Federal health-care systems: extending the services provided by maternal and child health nurses to mothers experiencing infant sleep problems resulted in health benefits to families at no significant increase in costs to society. However, this overall cost impact was driven by an increase in costs to (state-funded) providers of nurse services with a consequent saving to (largely federal-funded) providers of other health-care professional services (Hiscock et al. 2007). These "cost-shifting" patterns in resource use under different practice options can be assessed by reanalyzing evaluation results under alternative perspectives.

It is very common for the perspective of an evaluation to remain implicit, but an economic evaluation needs to be clear on perspective in order to identify the list of relevant costs and consequences that the evaluation needs to address. If an evaluation is being funded by and/or conducted for a government body or other organization, the perspective of the evaluation may well be specified in advance. For example, when the National Institute of Health and Clinical Excellence appraises health-care technologies for use in the NHS (England and Wales), the economic evaluation is required to take the perspective of the NHS and Personal Social Services (PSS) (National Institute for Health and Clinical Excellence 2008). In Canada, guidelines for evaluation of health technologies recommend the perspective of the publicly funded health-care system (Canadian Agency for Drugs and Technologies in Health 2006). This means that the costs and consequences for carers, patients' families, private business, and other government services (such as education) are not to be included in the evaluation.

## Evaluation context—measuring difference or difference in measurement?

Evaluation is a comparative endeavor. In an evaluation we seek to compare the performance of practice A and practice B. We conduct evaluation in order to decide whether A is better than B, where "better" is defined in terms of the consequences we wish to measure, relative to any change in costs.

In theory, to answer such comparative questions we do not need to measure the total impact that practice A has on consequences, nor the total impact that practice B has on consequences, only the *difference* in impact on these consequences between practice A and practice B. However, in practice we (or at least those sponsoring and/or participating in the evaluation) often do want to know the total impact of A and B, as well as the difference between them.

To consider this issue of measuring (only) difference or taking the difference in two measurements, imagine an evidence-based midwifery practice change that results (in a prior randomized controlled trial) in a reduction in the cesarean section rate of 5%. Do you want to know that practice A had a rate of 25% and B 20%? Would the decision be different if A were 15% and B 10%? What if A were 45% and B 40%? The question also applies to the costs side of the economic evaluation. If practice B costs $100 more per woman than A, do you also want to know that this is in the context of total costs for the episode of labor and delivery of $2,500 under practice A and $2,600 under practice B? Would your decision be different if the total cost of each practice were $500 for A and $600 for B?

It is actually very difficult to be sure, in advance, that the evaluation should *only* look at the difference between options under evaluation. However, this is exactly what evaluation methods, including economic evaluation methods, do. Economic evaluation is an efficiency-based concept and efficiency is a relative judgement on the incremental consequences (of A compared to B) when compared to the incremental investment required (of A compared to B).

## Identification of the costs and consequences relevant to the change in practice under evaluation

Once evaluation perspective and context have been agreed, the first step in economic evaluation is to write out a list of the all the costs and all the consequences that are relevant to the change in practice being evaluated. Relevant consequences include both all the potential positive outcomes and all the potential negative outcomes (or harms) from the change in practice; other chapters in this book discuss what these consequences might be and how we can measure them, therefore this chapter will focus on the costs side of the economic evaluation.

The list of costs relevant to a change in practice consists of two main groups of resources: those used to deliver the practice and those that are impacted later on *due to* the change in practice. Resources in economics are grouped into land (space), labor (people's time), and capital (bits of equipment) and this categorization is useful when drawing up the list of relevant costs. The first group of resources can include (depending on perspective): staff time (split by staff type or grade); patient time; clinic, theater, or office space; overheads such as electricity, catering, laundry, etc.; travel; use of large machines or equipment; consumables. The second group of resources includes the same type of resources, but this time we are thinking of those resources affected downstream from the change in practice, for example, due to reduced readmission rates, reduced treatment failure rates, or improved physical and mental health. The second group is easily overlooked and often difficult to measure, but can often be the source of potential cost savings (where follow-up costs are reduced due to the change in practice).

A final consideration in the identification of costs and consequences of practice change is the time horizon and physical or geographic horizon of the evaluation. In theory, a change in practice could have costs and consequences on all people passing through that practice setting now and in the future, and could have costs and consequences that permeate throughout time. In practice, evaluation (and economic evaluation) design requires some pragmatic decisions to be made around the length of time the evaluation will be conducted over and the breadth of possible beneficiaries or stakeholders that will be considered. For example, an evaluation of hospital-based postnatal care may decide to look only at outcomes for staff directly involved in the practice and the women and babies under their care (breadth of stakeholders) and to look at consequences up to 1 month after birth. Defining boundaries in this way does not deny the existence of other possible costs and consequences; rather, it makes an explicit distinction between those costs and consequences that we believe to be most central to the evaluation and those seen as more peripheral.

The peripheral costs and consequences also tend to be those that are harder to assign with certainty to the change in practice (e.g., how certain are we that a reduction in use of psychologist services by women in the year after birth is really due to a change in continuity of midwifery care in labor?). They can also be harder to measure, as they are difficult to predict in time and space (if practice change improves the self-sufficiency of patients, this should have knock-on benefits in other areas of their lives, but where and when should an evaluation measure to capture these predicted consequences?).

The importance of these boundary decisions will depend on the particular context of the evaluation. In general, boundary issues will be more critical for community-based health promotion practice than for more clinically oriented practice (Gold et al. 2007; Shiell et al. 2008).

## Measurement of costs and consequences

While the most noticeable changes to evaluation design from the incorporation of economic evaluation are on the costs side, there are often changes in the measurement of consequences. The inclusion of economic concepts can lead to a desire to include more patient-centered outcome measures in an evaluation, in order to get closer to a measure of the impact of practice change on the utility or happiness of those affected by that change. A CBA will use economic valuation techniques to estimate the value of benefits to key stakeholders (see below); this requires a description of expected consequences for that stakeholder in terms they can appreciate and understand. Evaluations that stop short of full CBA may still aim to measure consequences for multiple stakeholders in terms relevant to each group. This may be done in order to present a comprehensive picture of impacts on staff and patients, for example, in an evaluation of change in midwifery practice that promises improved outcomes for women but potential harm in terms of midwifery workload and burnout (McLachlan et al. 2008). Alternatively, patient-centered outcome measures such as quality-adjusted life years (QALYs) may be desired in order to derive evaluation outcomes in terms that are comparable to other health-care interventions (Canadian Agency for Drugs and Technologies in Health 2006; Drummond et al. 2005; National Institute for Health and Clinical Excellence 2008). QALYs are a composite health outcome measure that combine time (length of life, survival) and quality of life lived in that time (health-related quality of life, measured using one of the many available multi-attribute utility scales) (Drummond et al. 2005).

With a comprehensive list of identified costs and consequences from the first step of economic evaluation, the measurement of each item is simply a task of seeking evidence on the number of units of each identified item used as a result of the practice change (costs) or the number of units of change associated with the change in practice (consequences). All measurement is conducted in natural units, that is, the natural unit of measurement for each item. Therefore, staff time is measured in minutes or hours; travel in miles or kilometers;

consumables in number of items used; space in square meters; and so on. Consequences are measured as the change in proportion with adverse event X or outcome Y, or as the change in score on depression scale A or health-related quality of life scale B.

Complications arise, of course, when evidence is lacking on some of the items on the list of identified costs and consequences. This tends to happen more often for downstream costs and consequences, that is, those that are predicted to occur after a patient has experienced the change in practice (and commonly after they have left the practice setting). Evaluation can use "modeling" techniques to incorporate such predicted impacts on costs and consequences in a formal structure that brings together different evidence sources (Brennan & Akehurst 2000; Buxton 1997; Canadian Agency for Drugs and Technologies in Health 2006; Drummond et al. 2005; National Institute for Health and Clinical Excellence 2008; Philips et al. 2006). Such synthesis of different evidence sources is always possible, often inevitable, and best done with expert advice.

## Valuation of measured costs and consequences

The vast majority of economic evaluations in health care do not assign values to the measured change in the consequences of interest. Instead, the measured change in resource use is valued (in monetary terms) and compared to either a single measure of change in primary outcome (cost-effectiveness analysis or, when that measure is QALYs or similar, cost-utility analysis), or to multiple measures of change in all relevant outcomes (cost-consequences analysis) (Drummond et al. 2005). The limitation of these forms of economic evaluation is that there is usually a need for a separate final judgment over whether the additional benefits offered by a practice change are worth the additional costs involved. In some cases these economic evaluations can be conclusive, when they demonstrate either a "win-win" situation of increased benefits for no additional cost (COMET Study Group 2001; Hiscock et al. 2007) or indeed a "lose-lose" situation of a proposed change offering no increase in benefits but an increased cost (Wake et al. 2008).

Cost-benefit analysis (CBA) seeks to value the measured consequences in monetary terms and in order to do this requires use of an economic valuation technique. The two most common economic valuation techniques used in CBA in health care are willingness to pay and discrete choice experiments. Willingness to pay asks directly for an assessment of the value of (the consequences of) the practice change in monetary terms (Donaldson 1999); discrete choice experiments ask for choices between a series of practice scenarios and analyze the choices made to indirectly estimate the monetary value attached to the practice change under evaluation (Ryan 2000). Use of either technique requires the expert advice of an economist and can, depending on the technique used and how it is used, add significantly to evaluation costs. Both techniques have been used successfully in nursing and midwifery. One of the first studies to use willingness to pay was in the context of antenatal screening (Berwick & Weinstein 1985); more recent studies from the UK (Donaldson et al. 1998) and Australia (Taylor & Armour 2000) demonstrate its continued use both to assess women's values for health-care treatment options and within an economic evaluation (Hoddinott et al. 2009). Discrete choice experiments have been used fairly extensively across conception, pregnancy, and childbirth, particularly in the UK (Bishop et al. 2004; Hundley et al. 2001; Petrou & McIntosh 2009).

The valuation of all relevant costs in monetary terms is relatively straightforward, especially in health-care systems where there are already well-tested estimates of the cost of an item of resource use. Examples of these include the compilation of unit costs for health and social care (such as an hour of health visitor time, or a week of residential home care) in the England and Wales NHS (Curtis 2008) and casemix-based cost estimates of an episode of hospital care in many countries such as England and Wales (Department of Health 2008) and Australia (National Hospital Cost Data Collection 2008).

Any areas of disagreement over the most appropriate estimate to be used can be dealt with by testing the implications of using any given (set of) unit cost estimate(s) in a sensitivity analysis ("what if" analysis) of evaluation results (Drummond et al. 2005). For example, in a recent economic evaluation of a family doctor-led brief family intervention for child overweight/obesity in Australia, the intervention was associated with an average cost increase of Aus$4,094 for families. However, this estimate was based on parental time valued at the average Australian wage rate; if parents' time spent on the intervention were instead valued at zero (as only 9% of parents reported that they would otherwise be working), the additional cost associated with the intervention falls to Aus$1,562 (Wake et al. 2008).

Some items can be more complicated to measure than others, but there are usually well-tested methods around for dealing with these concerns. For example, large items of equipment may be used for multiple purposes and over a long equipment lifetime; the use associated with the practice under evaluation can be estimated as a fraction of all use of the equipment and costs apportioned over different uses. Equipment purchase costs can be spread appropriately over the expected equipment lifetime, including maintenance costs where appropriate.

Resource use that occurs later on in time than the main year of the evaluation needs to be valued in present value terms via the use of discounting (Drummond et al. 2005). There is some ongoing debate around whether consequences that happen in future years should be similarly discounted; most guidance calls for both future costs and consequences to be discounted at the same rate (3.5% in England and Wales; 5% in Canada) (Canadian Agency for Drugs and Technologies in Health 2006; National Institute for Health and Clinical Excellence 2008).

## Barriers to economic evaluation—ethics and research efficiency

### Economics and ethics in health-care evaluation

To many, the idea that the cost impact of a change in practice should have any influence on whether or not that practice change is seen as successful is unethical and abhorrent. It is important to state this concern upfront and deal with it now, rather than to pretend everything is rosy and stumble across it later on. The best response to this argument is presented by the late Professor Alan Williams, one of the founding fathers of health economics. He argued that doctors in a publicly funded health-care system have a dual role: to do the best for the individual patient and to do the best for all patients in the system, when it is known that not all needs can be met:

> The first part of this deliberation is concerned with clinical excellence, no matter what the costs. The second part is concerned with cost-effectiveness. Many doctors complain that the second part is really not part of ethical medical practice, which they believe enjoins them to do everything they can for each and every patient no matter what the costs. But one of the principles of medical ethics which I listed at the outset was to deal justly with patients.

Not counting the costs of your actions means not caring about the sacrifices that are imposed on others. In a resource-constrained system the "costs" of treating one patient are resources that might have been devoted to another patient, whose health will be worse by being deprived of them. Hence the need for prioritization, to ensure that what is sacrificed is less beneficial than what is done. This is what being cost-effective means.

(Williams 1998: p. 567)

## Staged evaluation (or the economic evaluation two step)—in theory and practice

A separate argument for excluding economic evaluation from the evaluation of practice change is that it is not worth looking at the impact of practice change on costs until we are certain that the practice change will have a positive impact on outcomes. This argument has intuitive appeal, especially when resources available for research, as for everything else, are limited (both in terms of the money available for evaluation and in terms of the availability of health economists). Including economic evaluation within an evaluation design will always add to research costs due to the need to search for and/or collect data on resource use as well as outcomes. If the economic evaluation requires modeling, inclusion of patient-centered outcome measures or monetary measures of benefit, these will add further to evaluation costs. Surely then it would be a cost-effective use of research funds to first evaluate the potential outcomes of practice change and only move on to an assessment of costs after benefit has been demonstrated? There are two counter-arguments: the process of decision making and the process of economic evaluation.

In the real world, timing is everything and (economic) evaluation will always be too early, until it is too late. Decision-making schedules rarely fit EBP and a staged evaluation inevitably falls victim to decision making prior to availability of economic evaluation results. If the intention is to postpone roll-out of beneficial practice change until a second-stage economic evaluation is completed, there are ethical issues around the feasibility of *not* acting on evidence of benefit. If the intention is to implement change and then reverse this should the economic evaluation show benefits are achieved at unacceptably high additional cost, there are serious questions around the (ir)reversibility of policy decisions.

A second argument against staged evaluation lies in the methods of economic evaluation, in that data collection processes for economic evaluation often need to run alongside the evaluation processes for collecting outcome data. If the methods for evaluation and economic evaluation are not separable, then there are few cost savings to be gained from removing economic evaluation and great additional costs to running a separate economic evaluation as a second-stage evaluation.

One often cited aspect of the cost of economic evaluation is the lack of available health economists. This is a valid argument, although often what is really meant is the lack of available health economics advice at zero cost. Links to local health economics advice can be found on the Internet via the International Health Economics Association and/or via the many national health economics groups (American Society of Health Economists, Health Economics Study Group (UK), Nordic Health Economists' Study Group, Canadian Health Economics Study Group, Australian Health Economics Society, etc.) as well as local consortia and university-based research groups. Access to economics advice should be part of the research support provided in any organization serious about improving the quality of EBP.

## Conclusion

Economic evaluation is a central and essential part of the assessment of EBP. We live in a resource-constrained world where every choice made has alternative paths that could have been taken, with alternative groups that could have benefited had we made a different choice. Choice is always costly, and we need to be more explicit in owning up to the fact that every decision we make has consequences not only for the patients that benefit (from our choice to go with a new, more expensive technology) but also for the patients that pay (by losing services cut to fund the new technology, or who would have been the recipient of those hours of nurse time that are now devoted to the patients receiving the new practice). Economic evaluation provides a well-developed framework within which to weigh up the differential costs and consequences arising from a change in practice. It will rarely answer the question for you, but will provide information in an explicit format for decision making. Whether decision makers want the information made so explicit is another question, but if we are to improve the quality and reach of EBP then we must all aim for an explicit consideration of not just the consequences of practice change but also of the additional resources required to effect such change (and where these resources come from).

## References

Berwick, D.M. & Weinstein M.C. (1985). What do patients value? Willingness-to-pay for ultrasound in normal pregnancy. *Medical Care*, 23, 881–893.

Bishop, A.J., Marteau, T.M., Armstrong, D. et al. (2004). Women and health care professionals' preferences for Down's Syndrome screening tests: A conjoint analysis study. *British Journal of Obstetrics and Gynaecology*, 111, 775–779.

Brennan, A. & Akehurst, R. (2000). Modelling in health economic evaluation: What is its place? What is its value? *PharmacoEconomics*, 17, 445–459.

Buxton, M. (1997). Modelling in economic evaluation: An unavoidable fact of life. *Health Economics*, 6, 217–227.

Canadian Agency for Drugs and Technologies in Health (2006). *Guidelines for the economic evaluation of health technologies: Canada*, 3rd ed. Ottawa: Canadian Agency for Drugs and Technologies in Health.

Comparative Obstetric Mobile Epidural Trial (COMET) Study Group UK (2001). Effect of low-dose mobile versus traditional epidural techniques on mode of delivery: A randomised controlled trial. *The Lancet*, 358, 19–23.

Cookson, R., Drummond, M., & Weatherly, H. (2009). Explicit incorporation of equity considerations into economic evaluation of public health interventions. *Health Economics, Policy and Law*, 4, 231–245.

Curtis, L. (Comp.) (2008). *Unit Costs of Health and Social Care 2008*. Canterbury: Personal Social Services Research Unit, University of Kent.

Department of Health (2008). *Reference Costs (2006–2007)*. London: The Stationery Office.

Donaldson, C. (1999). Valuing the benefits of publicly-provided health care: Does "ability to pay" preclude the use of "willingness to pay." *Social Science and Medicine*, 49, 551–563.

Donaldson, C., Hundley, V., & Mapp, T. (1998). Willingness to pay: A method for measuring preferences for maternity care? *Birth*, 25, 32–39.

Drummond, M.F., Sculpher, M.J., Torrance, G.W., O'Brien, B.J., & Stoddart, G.L. (2005). *Methods for the Economic Evaluation of Health Care Programmes*, 3rd ed. Oxford: Oxford University Press.

Gold, M.R., Siegel, J.E., Russell, L.B., & Weinstein, M.C. (1996). *Cost-Effectiveness in Health and Medicine*. New York: Oxford University Press.

Gold, L., Shiell, A., Hawe, P., Riley, T., Rankin, B., & Smithers, P. (2007). The costs of a community based intervention to promote maternal health. *Health Education Research*, 22, 648–657.

Hiscock, H., Bayer, J., Gold, L., Hampton, A., Ukoumunne, O., & Wake, M. (2007). Improving infant sleep and maternal mental health: a cluster randomised trial. *Archives of Disease in Childhood*, 92, 952–958.

Hoddinott, P., Britten, J., Prescott, G.J., Tappin, D., Ludbrook, A., & Godden, D.J. (2009). Effectiveness of policy to provide breastfeeding groups (BIG) for pregnant and breastfeeding mothers in primary care: Cluster randomised trial. *British Medical Journal*, 338, a3026.

Hundley, V., Ryan, M., & Graham, W. (2001). Assessing women's preferences for intrapartum care. *Birth*, 28, 254–263.

Jefferson, T., Demicheli, V., & Mugford, M. (2000). *Elementary Economic Evaluation in Health Care*, 2nd ed. London: BMJ Books.

McLachlan, H., Forster, D., Davey, M-A. et al. (2008). COSMOS: COmparing Standard Maternity care with One-to-one midwifery Support: A randomised controlled trial. *BMC Pregnancy and Childbirth*, 8, 35.

National Hospital Cost Data Collection (2008). *Cost Report Round 11 (2006–2007)*. Canberra: Commonwealth Department of Health and Ageing in conjunction with the States and Territories.

National Institute for Health and Clinical Excellence (2008). *Guide to the Methods of Technology Appraisal*. London: National Institute for Health and Clinical Excellence.

Petrou, S. & McIntosh, E. (2009). Women's preferences for attributes of first-trimester miscarriage management: A stated preference discrete-choice experiment. *Value Health*, 12, 551–559.

Philips, Z., Bojke, L., Sculpher, M., Claxton, K., & Golder, S. (2006). Good practice guidelines for decision-analytic modelling in health technology assessment. *PharmacoEconomics*, 24, 355–371.

Ryan, M. (2000). Using conjoint analysis to elicit preferences for health care. *British Medical Journal*, 320, 1530–1533.

Shiell, A., Donaldson, C., Mitton, C., & Currie, G. (2002) Health economic evaluation: A glossary is presented on terms of health economic evaluation. Definitions are suggested for the more common concepts and terms. *Journal of Epidemiology and Community Health*, 56, 85–88.

Shiell, A., Hawe, P., & Gold, L. (2008) Complex interventions or complex systems? Implications for health economic evaluation. *British Medical Journal*, 336, 1281–1283.

Taylor, S.J. & Armour, C.L. (2000). Measurement of consumer preference for treatments used to induce labour: A willingness to pay approach. *Health Expectations*, 3, 203–216.

Wake, M., Gold, L., McCallum, Z., Gerner, B., & Waters, E. (2008). Economic evaluation of a primary care trial to reduce weight gain in overweight/obese children: The LEAP trial. *Ambulatory Pediatrics*, 8, 336–341.

Williams A. (1998). Medicine, economics, ethics and the NHS: A clash of cultures? *Health Economics*, 7, 565–568.

# Chapter 9

# Sustaining evidence-based practice systems and measuring the impacts

*Barbara Davies, Dominique Tremblay, and Nancy Edwards*

---

**Key learning points**

- Sustainability of evidence-based practice is a vital consideration to maintain or increase improvements in the provision of quality health care and patient outcomes and to avoid erosion or decay of a practice.
- Evidence-based practices require ongoing attention to changes in an organization or practice setting as well as watchful monitoring for new evidence and priority outcomes.
- The National Health Service sustainability model includes 10 factors clustered around the dimensions of process, staff, and organization. Other determinants include the political and power dimension, the need for priority setting, and a common language for stakeholders.
- Emerging promising practices for sustainability include a "yes we can attitude," individual and collective reflective practice, leadership, and performance evaluation.

---

## Introduction

This chapter includes definitions and models about sustainability to assist health care providers and decision-makers to design and sustain evidence-based practice (EBP) and measure its ongoing impact. Five strategies based on the literature and our experience for attaining more sustainable EBP are outlined: developing a "yes we can" attitude; interprofessional reflective practice; individual, multilevel, and collective leadership; evidence generation and use; and performance evaluation. The creation of broad-based indicators to support and measure the sustainability of health care changes are emphasized along with quantitative, qualitative, and participatory approaches to evaluation. Two exemplars are described to illustrate issues and approaches to sustainability planning in cancer care and long-term database development in perinatal care. Future recommendations for sustainability-oriented EBP and research are described.

## The need for and concept of "sustainability" of EBP change

Efforts to sustain the implementation of EBP changes are imperative; otherwise any improvements made to practice by health care providers may be lost after the completion of a project (Argentine Episiotomy Trial Collaborative Group 1993). Sustainability is defined as "the degree to which an innovation continues to be used after initial efforts to secure adoption are completed" (Rogers 2003) or "when new ways of working become the norm" (Maher et al. 2007). In order to prevent the fading or decay of short-term improvements, it is vital to continue to maintain or adapt an EBP and to evaluate its integrity and sustainability. There are no quick fixes for dealing with sustainability. A "vigilant diagnostic approach" to monitoring both supporting and threatening factors over the time period when the EBP should be encouraged is recommended (Buchanan et al. 2007: p. 23.)

## Maintaining the integrity of EBP

### Adaptation due to changes in the organization

Maintaining the integrity of an EBP and the active ingredients of what make an EBP work is straightforward when the situation remains constant. However, in health care systems, change is the norm with the dual dynamics of changes in both organizational factors and the emergence of new evidence. With respect to the organizational perspective, factors such as the availability of new types of health care providers or availability of new equipment may influence the integrity of an EBP. Thus, from a sustainability perspective, it is highly likely that adaptation of an EBP will be required over time. Periodic evaluations will be important to determine whether subsequent organizational modifications or changes in the practice environment influence use of an EBP and whether this positively or negatively has an impact on outcomes. For complex interventions, it is recommended that the function and process of an intervention be standardized but not the specific components (Hawe et al. 2004).

For example, with respect to the provision of continuous support for women during childbirth, a meta-analysis of 16 trials involving 13,391 women in 11 countries found that women randomized to receive continuous support were more likely to have spontaneous vaginal births and were less likely to report dissatisfaction with their childbirth experiences (Hodnett et al. 2007). Of note was that support appeared to be more effective when provided by women who were not part of the hospital staff. The active function and process ingredients of this complex intervention are the theory-based aspects of the provision of emotional support, comfort measures, information and advocacy. Specific support behaviors are tailored to an individual woman's context, such as her culture, attendance at prenatal education, and other available support from a spouse or family member. The meta-analysis concluded that "all women should have support throughout labour and birth" yet it is still evident that "in hospitals worldwide that continuous support during labour has become the exception rather than the routine" (Hodnett et al. 2007).

Maintaining the integrity of an EBP such as the provision of continuous support for women during childbirth is influenced by organizational barriers such as the use of a unit's central fetal monitoring system, which encourages charting and monitoring outside of the woman's room (Graham et al. 2004). Thus, we recommend that care providers and decision-makers regularly consider organizational factors that may influence the active ingredients and the integrity of EBP. As stated by Denis et al. (2002), complex interventions are not a "thing" with fixed boundaries but include a "hard core" of its irreducible elements (e.g., elements of the provision of support during labor) and a "soft periphery" of the structures and systems that need to be in place for sustainability.

# Adaptation due to the emergence of new evidence

Ongoing systems are required to inform health care providers and decision-makers about new evidence and EBPs, so that they can selectively apply, adapt, or discontinue the implementation of an EBP. For example, the ongoing "sustained" implementation of an outdated clinical best practice guideline is not advisable. Systems need to be put in place to find and appraise the results of promising new research evidence; retrieve and appraise new and updated guidelines; examine patient preferences for EBP options; obtain input about clinician's experiences implementing guidelines; and learn about other emerging EBPs and contextual influences. A leader from a high-performing health care organization explains that sustainability is a challenge because their "just do it culture" results in many concurrent improvement activities (Baker et al. 2008). This leader also highlights that there is "a continuing need to prioritize project commitments systematically, to divest those projects that produce marginal outcomes and to complete priority projects before engaging in new ones" (Baker et al. 2008: pp. 260–261). This quote illustrates that health care providers and leaders need to be active and not passive recipients of new evidence (knowledge) and need to collectively determine the relative advantage of new EBP. From a sustainability perspective, selective monitoring of priority outcomes of concurrent initiatives as well as previously established EBP is required.

## Sustainability models

Although 11 of 31 models about knowledge translation describe a separate step subsequent to evaluation entitled maintaining change or sustaining ongoing knowledge use (Graham et al. 2007), very few studies have been conducted about the determinants of sustainability. Only 2 of 1000 sources screened in a systematic review of the diffusion of innovations in health services organizations mentioned the term sustainability (Greenhalgh et al. 2005). Furthermore, sustainability is not a common key word indexed in evidence-based textbooks such as Evidence-Based Nursing (DiCenso et al. 2005) or Using Evidence (Nutley et al. 2007). However, the term *sustainable* is frequently used by policy-makers and politicians in Canada, UK, USA, and other countries as they strive to develop and maintain "sustainable" health care services and programs for the public.

## Priority setting for sustainability

How might priorities be set from a sustainability perspective? One research team has recently proposed a new priority setting conceptual framework to help address the complex decision-making required to sustain health care systems that are constantly challenged by increasing service demands and new technology (Sibbald et al. 2009). The framework was derived from three empirical studies and is intended for decision-makers of clinical programs, hospitals, regional authorities, or governments. The framework includes 10 elements in two clusters of process and outcome concepts. The *process* concepts are stakeholder engagement, use of explicit process, information management, consideration of values and context, and revision or appeal mechanisms. The *outcome* concepts are improved stakeholder understanding, shifted priorities and/ or reallocated resources, improved decision-making quality, stakeholder acceptance and satisfaction, and positive externalities (e.g., media and accreditation). This model is useful because it articulates defined process outcomes, acknowledges the importance of values and context, and provides a common language for stakeholders to discuss contentious issues. However, the model does not include the measurement of health outcomes such as morbidity, mortality, quality of life, or patient/client satisfaction. How will decision-makers and health care providers decide when health outcomes are marginal or when to stop an EBP and test out a new approach? Ongoing evaluation of this promising priority setting model with concurrent health outcome analyses is a potential area of research.

## The NHS sustainability model

Despite the limited research about sustainability, the National Health Service (NHS) in the UK has been a leader in the code-velopment of a sustainability model with and for the NHS by frontline teams, administrators, and experts from industry and academia (Maher et al. 2007). The model was developed using a multifaceted approach based on the change management litera-ture, and an analysis of focus group discussions with health care experts and 250 NHS staff (Maher et al., personal communica-tion). Initially, over 100 factors were identified. Subsequently these factors were ranked and regression analyses were conducted to develop a predictive scoring system. To date, the authors report receiving extensive feedback about the utility of the model, which is currently being used in a US-based study (Maher et al., personal communication).

The model includes 10 factors clustered in three major dimensions of process, staff, and organization (Maher et al. 2007). A strength of this model is that is includes the measurement of health outcomes as an important factor, a limitation of the previously described priority setting model (Sibbald et al. 2009). Developers suggest that this model is useful for planning specific sustained EBP changes at the team, organizational or community level. Using the model during the initial implementation process is recommended by the authors to avoid sustainability failure, which is estimated at 33% for health care initiatives and 70% for organizational changes (Maher et al. 2007). The model can be used as a diagnostic tool to identify potential barriers to sustainability. A leaders' guide is available which describes practical tips (NHS Institute for Innovation and Improvement 2007). An excel spreadsheet can readily be downloaded at no cost from the National Leadership and Innovation Agency for Healthcare in the UK (2009) to assess factors thought to influence sustainability. The following list includes the NHS model elements and their corresponding indicators for self-assessment by leaders and teams attempting to design sustainable health care change. Further details to assess each indicator are included in the model and guide. In the following section, each indicator is described, as quoted from Maher et al. (2007).

### Process factors

- *Benefits beyond helping patients: The change improves efficiency and makes jobs easier*
- *Credibility of the evidence: Benefits of the change are immediately obvious, supported by evidence and believed by stakeholders*
- *Adaptability of improved process: The process can be adapted to other organizational changes and there is a system for continually improving the process*
- *Effectiveness of the system to monitor progress: There is a system in place to identify evidence of progress, monitor progress, act on it and communicate results*

### Staff factors

- *Staff involvement and training to sustain the process: Staff have been involved from the beginning of change and adequately trained to sustain the improved process*
- *Staff behaviours toward sustaining the change: Staff feel empowered as part of the change process and believe the improvement will be sustained*
- *Senior leadership engagement: Organizational leaders take responsibility for efforts to sustain the change process, Staff generally share information with, and actively seek advice from, the leader*
- *Clinical leadership engagement: Clinical leaders take responsibility for efforts to sustain the change process, Staff generally share information with, and actively seek advice from, the leader*

### Organizational factors

- *Fit with the organisation's strategic aims and culture: There is a history of successful sustainability and improvement goals are consistent with the organizations strategic aims*
- *Infrastructure for sustainability: Staff, facilities and equipment, job descriptions, policies, procedures and communication systems are appropriate for sustaining the improved process*

The NHS model developers recommend that teams concentrate on factors with lower scores and thus room for improvement. Figure 9.1 displays an example of hypothetical scores for sustainability factors. The hypothetical data indicate that the score for the factor "effectiveness of the system to monitor progress" was low. In this scenario, teams, providers and stakeholders should identify relevant data, access the data and communicate the results to patients/clients, staff and the regional or national health care system.

Future research needs to test the relative weights of this scoring system in different applications and settings and to prospectively study whether the implementation of sustainability action plans arising from an assessment using the model, improves success rates and outcomes. However, sustainability planning is only one important aspect. The ongoing adaptation of EBP that is required due to organizational changes and new emerging evidence is perhaps the more urgent research needed since it is disheartening for clinicians,

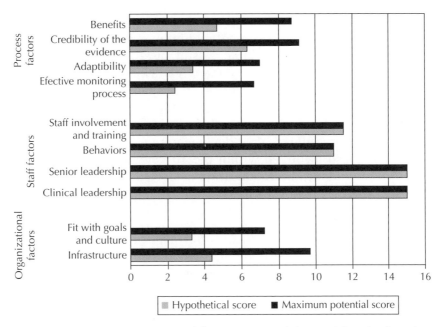

**Figure 9.1** Score for the elements of the NHS sustainability model—using hypothetical data in an accessible excel spreadsheet from the UK National Leadership and Innovation Agency for Healthcare.
Adapted from Maher et al. (2007); http://www.wales.nhs.uk/sitesplus/829/page/36527.

managers, and senior administrators to see erosions in health care after successful changes were made in short-term EBP projects. Future research needs to test whether or not this NHS sustainability model or a priority setting sustainability framework or a combination of models improves and sustains outcomes over the long term.

It is interesting to review the scoring mechanisms of the NHS sustainability model and note that the potential for the highest scores as ranked by the experts and focus group participants (Maher et al. 2007) are for the senior and clinical leadership dimensions of the model. These higher proposed scores for leadership are consistent with the results of a Canadian study to determine factors related to the sustained implementation of nursing guidelines (Davies et al. 2006). Leadership, defined as "recognizable role models, leaders, champions or administrative support," was the only significant predictor explaining 47% of the variance of how strongly a guideline permeated the organization 2 years after the original implementation (Davies et al. 2006). Examining the critical factors apparent in sustainability failures is just as important as determining the factors in successful sustainability. With respect to the previously mentioned nursing guideline implementation study, we found that in the 16 health care organizations that did not sustain guideline implementation, that there was no ongoing staff education and no integration of the guideline recommendations in policies, procedures, or e-documentation. Of note, these two factors are also identified within the 10 key factors in the NHS sustainability model. Staff education is labeled as training and involvement where as policy/documentation is labeled as infrastructure (Maher et al. 2007).

One other variable that is not explicit in the sustainability model but that has been reported in the literature is the political and power dimension (Buchanan et al. 2007; Davies & Edwards 2009). Attention needs to be paid to the power, influences, and support of stakeholders (Edwards & Roelofs 2006). The need for "intense" sustainability efforts that can buffer changing political and economic factors has been described graphically by a leader of a high-performing health care organization as "hurricane-proofing the change initiatives to protect against the inevitable next cycle of budget reductions and staff cuts" (Baker et al. 2008: p. 205).

## Strategies for more sustainable EBP

While models for sustainability provide useful guidance to plan for the implementation of future EBP, there are also some emerging promising practices. In this section we describe specific evidence-based strategies for sustaining EBP improvements.

### (1) Developing a "yes, we can attitude"
The importance of rhetoric and opinion leaders' positive discourse has been found to play a central role for innovation to succeed (Akrich et al. 2002). This positive approach highlights the necessity to use strategies beyond "barriers management" that has been a major focus in the EBP literature. A barriers-oriented approach can lead to inertia (Marchionni & Richer 2007), particularly if there are long-standing issues. Improving sustainability requires building positive thinking and celebrating small wins through a stepwise evolution. Appreciative inquiry is a social process that builds a

positive dialogue among stakeholders to rediscover their aspirations and to use these aspirations to reach collective goals (Cooperrider & Whitney 2000). Appreciative inquiry has been described as a change philosophy that shifts the discourse from a focus on deficits to an emphasis on the potential of individuals and organizations (Lind & Smith 2008). The appreciative approach offers a capacity-building orientation to implementing EBPs, which may be a stimulus for sustained improvement.

### (2) Interprofessional reflective practice

Based on largely theoretical evidence (Duffy 2007; Mann et al. 2007), there is a growing body of literature suggesting pragmatic linkages between reflective practice and long-term EBP (Mantzoukas & Watkinson 2008; McWilliam 2007; Paget 2001; Rolfe 2005; Watkins et al. 2004). Reflective practice is the act of interrogating the efficacy of daily practice to learn from professional experience (Schön 1983). Reflective practice is both an individual and a collective action that introduces a mode of being aware of the strengths and weaknesses of practice. This approach has been credited with empowering the practitioner to enact desirable and effective practice (Duffy 2007; Sandywell 1996). Reflective practice discussions provide a deliberative forum for clarifying, analyzing, and using evidence. EBP and reflective activities increase sustainability in creating a space for appropriation of new knowledge as an emerging internal process rather than an imposed external innovation. The former provides the foundation for research-based clinical practice and the latter allows the professional assessment and reassessment of clinical EBPs and routines. As professionals are more receptive to innovation emerging from their internal dynamics rather than those imposed by an external imperative (Ferlie et al. 2005), EBP and reflective practice create the synergy for sustainable change "integrating science push and demand pull" occurring within the process of social interaction (McWilliam et al. 2009: p. 7).

### (3) Leadership: Individual, multilevel, and collective

The literature on innovation clearly demonstrates the importance of individual leadership for EBP implementation (Akrich et al. 2002; Berwick 2003; Rogers 2003). Even with the scarcity of research about the determinants of sustainability, we can anticipate that leadership is a cornerstone for sustained EBP. Indeed, in a secondary analysis of qualitative data to investigate factors that contributed to sustaining (or not) the use of clinical guidelines in professional nursing practice, a different pattern of leadership was found in organizations that sustained guideline implementation (Gifford et al. 2006). Three broad leadership strategies emerged as central to successfully implementing and sustaining guidelines in nursing: (1) facilitating individual staff to use the guidelines, (2) creating a positive milieu of best practices, and (3) influencing organizational structures and processes (Gifford et al. 2006). Specific leadership activities included providing support, being accessible and visible, communicating well, reinforcing goals and philosophy, influencing change, role modeling commitment, ensuring education and policy, monitoring clinical outcomes, and supporting the development of clinical champions. This study illustrates the importance of leaders' multilevel involvement to support sustained behavior change for professional practice.

From a broader perspective, focusing on health system pluralism, the dynamics of collective leadership could appear to be a master piece for sustainable EBP change. Pluralistic organizations are characterized by multiple objectives with competing values, diffuse power and knowledge-based work processes (Denis et al. 2007). The complexity of pluralistic organizations calls for the development of unified collective leadership rather than individuals imposing separate visions for EBP.

## (4) Evidence and sustainability

The approach used to generate and apply evidence to health care systems may contribute to enhanced use of evidence by decision-makers (Glasgow & Emmons 2007; Landry et al. 2003). EBP sustainability initiatives need to address the limitations of linear (A → B) diffusion models. Evidence production and use involves different networks of health care providers, each having their own values, interests, priorities, dynamics, means of communication, objectives, and boundary management (Best et al. 2008). We suggest that evidence application that spans traditional boundaries for health care delivery may not only support sustained use of evidence, but also generate new evidence gaps that will need to be addressed by teams of researchers who are also willing to cross their network boundaries. Research priorities identified considering contextual factors may be more likely to reflect the complexity of the practice environment, yielding health services research that is more relevant for decision-making and interprofessional practice (Glasgow & Emmons 2007).

## (5) Performance evaluation

Performance evaluation has a role to support change and ensure sustainability (Potvin & Golberg 2006). A broad-based approach is recommended to identify and measure the wide range of impacts that EBP may have at a particular level of a health care system (clinical, organizational, and governance). Indicator identification should occur before implementation begins. Sustainability indicators are essential building blocks in evidence-based planning, management, and monitoring processes.

Good sustainability indicators must be easy to understand, as well as clinically and economically feasible to measure. Based on our experience and the literature, some of the benefits from developing and using good indicators include:

- More timely decision-making, which may help reduce risks and/or costs,
- Identification of emerging risks and or conflicting issues that may compromise sustainability,
- Identification of impacts, to allow for timely corrective action when needed,
- Setting clear benchmarks for ongoing performance measurement,
- Greater public accountability, that is, providing credible information for the public and other stakeholders,
- Providing the means to monitor for continuous quality improvement,
- Earlier identification of unanticipated adverse effects or unexpected benefits, thus identifying limits and opportunities.

## A suggested development process for indicators that will be sustainable

At the outset, it is important to recognize that different levels of health indicators are required for health planning and regulation processes. For example, system-level cancer care performance indicators in Ontario, Canada, were developed in the context of a long-standing health strategy and planning process based on best-available evidence (Greenberg et al. 2005). In this case, focusing on sustainability indicators can help improve data sources, monitoring functions, and reporting processes. Literature on the sustainability of innovation and performance in health services (Agency for Healthcare Research and Quality 2008; Baker et al. 2008; Greenberg et al. 2005; Pluye et al. 2004; Sicotte et al. 1998) suggests a step-by-step process to maximize the coherence among evidence, professional routines, and organizational culture. Based on this literature, we have generated Figure 9.2. This process for developing sustainable indicators is not linear. The fundamental base is the development of a collaborative approach between researchers and care providers followed by the identification of indicators and data sources. The third step concentrates on evaluation and feedback for practice adjustment.

## Criteria for selecting sustainability indicators

The main criteria for selecting sustainability indicators in health should be:

- **Relevance** of the indicator to the selected issue for stakeholders' long-term objectives,
- **Feasibility** of obtaining and analyzing the needed information in a way that informs timely decision-making in order to stabilize practice around the desired outcomes,

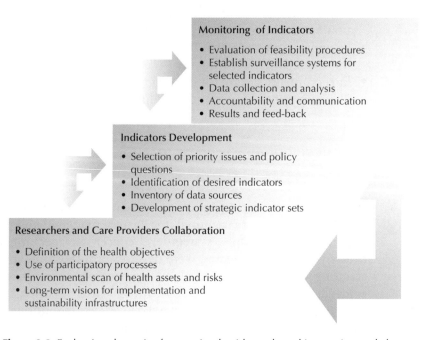

**Monitoring of Indicators**
- Evaluation of feasibility procedures
- Establish surveillance systems for selected indicators
- Data collection and analysis
- Accountability and communication
- Results and feed-back

**Indicators Development**
- Selection of priority issues and policy questions
- Identification of desired indicators
- Inventory of data sources
- Development of strategic indicator sets

**Researchers and Care Providers Collaboration**
- Definition of the health objectives
- Use of participatory processes
- Environmental scan of health assets and risks
- Long-term vision for implementation and sustainability infrastructures

**Figure 9.2** Evaluation dynamics for sustained evidence-based innovation and change

- **Credibility** of the information and reliability for users,
- **Clarity** and ability to be understood by users, and
- **Comparability** over time and across jurisdictions or regions.

In summary, ongoing responsible decision-making by health managers needs to be based on reliable information and well-defined indicators. In addition to supporting health planning and monitoring processes, indicators are also important tools for communication. Sustainability of EBPs calls for new forms of problem solving and analysis, in which feedback is injected into decision-making at each level of the health system (clinical, managerial, and strategic). Here sustainability of EBP is not the end point of a change but rather a messy trajectory, of constant efforts to adapt global recommendations from evidence to local contexts and reconfigure the patterns of day-to day practices.

Changes (both positive and negative) may arise from the sustained implementation of an EBP and are not necessarily predictable. Thus, it is important not to rely exclusively on pre-established measurement scales. These need to be complemented with process and qualitative means to examine and understand the unforeseen (Bowman et al. 2008). The process of designing sustainability-related indicators can be contentious particularly if the indicators lack clinical credibility with the health care providers or the monitoring approach is punitive (Buchanan et al. 2007: p. 270). Frontline clinical perspectives on the selection of indicators, data collection methods, and how the data should be interpreted may differ substantially from managerial or strategic perspectives. From a sustainability perspective, it is thus very important to use an inclusive approach to performance evaluation.

## Exemplars and issues around the sustainability of EBP systems

Although there is limited research on the determinants of sustainability and the measurement of the long-term impacts of EBP, we are involved in two long-term EBP initiatives. Our experience illustrates issues in sustainability planning and measurement. Exemplars include an interprofessional collaborative cancer care program and a 15-year program for the development of a regional perinatal database to monitor EBP.

## An exemplar: interprofessional collaborative practices among cancer teams

The regional cancer network in Montérégie (Réseau Cancer Montérégie), a socio-health region in Québec, planned to expand interprofessional collaboration among nurses, doctors, and other care providers (pharmacists, nutritionists, and social workers) working in cancer teams.

Although the benefits of interprofessional collaboration for users, for providers, and for organizations are well supported by high-quality evidence (Health Professions Regulatory Advisory Council, 2008; Oandasan et al. 2006; Sitzia et al. 2006), many professionals pay lip-service to the premise of collaborative practice (Thornhill et al. 2008). The challenges of sustaining new patterns of professional practice emerging from evidence-based recommendations were numerous when a program was developed to translate evidence-based recommendations from the Registered Nurses' Association of Ontario (RNAO 2006) best practice guidelines about collaborative practice among nursing teams in day-to-day practice. The program is nurse-led and uses recommendations of EBP guidelines (RNAO 2002, 2006, 2008) and other sources of evidence (Association of Ontario Health Centers [AOHC] 2007; Brazil et al. 2003).

A sustainability plan was implemented at the outset. It was based on the premise that a trusting and supportive network, planned from the beginning of the project, would foster sustainability throughout a reconfiguration of relationships between stakeholders. The supportive network helped to ensure mentorship by expert clinician and managers, to identify barriers, to find negotiated solutions in a step-wise manner, and to support long-standing practice renewal. Local leaders, recognized for their clinical expertise and their abilities to mobilize their colleagues, helped to reinforce the linkages between practitioners and expert clinicians.

The program has found that general recommendations from evidence, such as those contained in best practice guidelines, need to be adapted to the contextual dynamics to become routinized. Barriers to sustainable practice changes included a lack of consensus about the nature of collaborative practice and competition among professionals that inevitably emerges when collaboration leads to new divisions of labor (Reay et al. 2003). The need for local leaders who would continue to be involved in the project after the initial educational stage of implementation (Thomas et al. 1998; Wensing & Grol 2005) and the need for managers who could help to resolve tensions around turf protection were identified as supports for sustaining these EBP changes.

Evaluative research to determine the impact on patient care is being conducted. The program illustrates challenges in the application of sustainability planning processes integrated with the measurement of outcomes for improved practice with a partnership approach. Long-term follow-up of the routinization of the new practices, roles, and responsibilities will be important in monitoring whether this sustainability plan is successful or not.

## An exemplar: long-term regional EBP perinatal database

The Perinatal Partnership Program is a collaborative intersector, interprofessional network of 37 organizations providing perinatal care in hospitals, health departments, community agencies, academic institutions, and private practice in a region of Ontario, Canada. During a period of widespread budget cuts, staff layoffs, and hospital closures, the board of directors of the network realized that one of the most valuable components to fund even under extreme financial duress was the Niday Perinatal Database, named after a visionary nursing leader Dr Patricia Niday. The provision of timely data was and continues to be a priority for a network with the vision that "child-bearing families, women and babies receive accessible, evidence-based care consistently throughout the region" (Perinatal Partnership Program 2008). After 10 years of development and refinement, this database was selected to be a central model for the whole province incorporating data from 93% of 121,932 births (hospital/home) (Ontario Perinatal Partnership Program 2006).

The database is currently a web-based system funded by the Government of Ontario. Data may be entered directly from sites or uploaded from individual hospital or community-based databases. This flexibility allows individual hospitals to maintain their own unique data information systems and also participate in regional and provincial programs. Data quality is addressed on a regular basis with the help of a web-based user and dictionary guide. Staff at each participating hospital receives ongoing training. Online error identification is built into the systems.

Sustainability of practice changes and long-term trends are highlighted with 5-year graphs by region and type of institution (teaching hospital versus community hospital). Examples of EBP of current concern are the rising rates of induction and cesarean section. Detailed data are provided to each participating organization about their own rates with summary charts benchmarking similar types of settings (e.g., teaching, large community, and small community hospitals). An annual report includes additional text summarizing relevant research evidence such as systematic reviews and guideline recommendations highlighting EBPs. In the most recent report, there is a spotlight on reducing cesarean birth with referenced recommendations about intensive data feedback and strong departmental leadership (Perinatal Partnership Program 2008).

A cautionary note is warranted about sustainability surveillance systems like the Niday Perinatal Database. Surveillance systems are largely set up to provide timely data that monitors critical changes to population health. Epidemiological approaches to measuring disease outcomes provide some of the underpinnings for what gets measured and how data gets reported. The development of surveillance systems takes substantial commitment and many years of effort and consensus building on underlying taxonomies and indicators (definitions and measurement). Establishing a smooth chain of surveillance reporting and timely analysis requires solid capacity for each link in the chain.

However, that which makes surveillance systems rigorous and informative is arguably their weakness. They are generally not designed to pick up nuanced changes that may be seen by those working on the front lines. In a study by Meagher-Stewart et al. (in press) for instance, public health nurses described adverse social changes that were being experienced by those living in poverty as a result of implementing provincial policy on health care restructuring. The public health nurses' observations were astute, but the nurses had no means to report these observations as they did not "fit" with the existing surveillance system indicators. Interestingly, such observations may provide important insights into early modifications that need to be made by those implementing change processes. In the case of policy change, frontline observations may assist with the identification of differential effects on subpopulations, providing guidance on regulations that are required or enforcement strategies that might be needed. Thus, existing surveillance systems may not demonstrate the unintended (and in particular unwanted) effects of new EBPs or policies. The insights of frontline practitioners and managers may complement the aggregated data from existing surveillance systems and help identify unintended effects of change. This can help to ensure that the evidence-based changes which are being introduced should be sustained.

## Conclusion

Sustaining EBPs and measuring their impacts are essential for improving the quality of health care systems and improving patient outcomes. Careful attention is needed to maintain the integrity of an EBP, as practice may need to be adapted due to changes in the organizational environment and/or the emergence of new evidence. Available sustainability models are multifactorial and include process, staff, organizational and outcome-based elements. To date, little research has been conducted from a sustainability perspective, yet sustainable EBP and health care systems are considered important by policy-makers and the public (Shediac-Rizkallah & Bone 1998; Sibbald 2009). Strategies for more sustainable EBP are recommended which include attention to attitudes, interprofessional practice, leadership, and broad-based indicator development. We recommend that future research use a theory-based approach simultaneously studying priority setting, processes for health care from an interprofessional perspective, and selected patient outcomes.

## References

Agency for Healthcare Research and Quality. (2008). Will it work here? A decisionmaker's guide to adopting innovations. Retrieved March 16, 2009, from http://www.innovations.ahrq.gov/resources/InnovationAdoptionGuide.pdf.

Akrich, M., Callon, M., & Latour, B. (2002). The key to success in innovation part II. The art of choosing good spokespersons. *International Journal of Innovation Management*, 6(2), 207–225.

Argentine Episiotomy Trial Collaborative Group. (1993). Routine vs selective episiotomy: A randomised controlled trial. *The Lancet*, 342(8886–8887), 1517–1518.

Association of Ontario Health Centers (AOHC). (2007). Building better teams: A toolkit for strengthening teamwork in community health centres. Retrieved July 25, 2009, from http://www.aohc.org/aohc/index.aspx?CategoryID=24&lang=en-CA.

Baker, G.R., MacIntosh-Murray, A., Porcellato, C., Dionne, L., Stelmacovich, K., & Born, K. (2008). *High Performing Healthcare Systems: Delivering Quality by Design*. Toronto Canada: Longwoods.

Berwick, D.M. (2003). Disseminating innovations in health care. *JAMA: The Journal of the American Medical Association*, 289, 1969–1975.

Best, A., Trochim, W.K., Haggerty, J., Moor, G., & Norman, C.D. (2008). Systems thinking for knowledge integration: New models for policy-research collaboration. In: L. McKee, E. Ferlie, & P. Hyde (eds) *Organizing and Reorganizing. Power and Change in Health Care Organizations*. New York: Palgrave Macmillan.

Bowman, C.C., Sobo, E.J., Asch, S.M., & Gifford, A.L. (2008). Measuring persistence of implementation: QUERI series. *Implementation Science*, 3(1), 21.

Brazil, K., Whelan, T., O'Brien, M. et al. (2003). *Coordinating Supportive Cancer Care in the Community—Final Report*. Hamilton, Ontario: The Supportive Cancer Care Research Unit.

Buchanan, D.A., Fitzgerald, L., & Ketley, D. (2007). *The Sustainability and Spread of Organizational Change: Modernizing Healthcare*. New York: Routledge.

Cooperrider, D.L. & Whitney, D. (2000). A positive revolution in change: Appreciative inquiry. Retrieved April 7, 2009, from http://appreciativeinquiry.case.edu/uploads/whatisai.pdf.

Davies, B. & Edwards, N. (2009). The action cycle: Sustain knowledge use. In: S. Strauss, J. Tetroe, & I. Graham (eds) *Knowledge to Translation in Health Care: Moving from Evidence to Practice*. Oxford: Wiley-Blackwell and BMJ, pp. 165–173.

Davies, B., Edwards, N., Ploeg, J., Virani, T., Skelly, J., & Dobbins, M. (2006). *Determinants of the Sustained Use of Research Evidence in Nursing: Final Report*. Ottawa, Ontario, Canada: Canadian Health Services Research Foundation & Canadian Institutes for Health Research. Retrieved December July 25, 2009, from http://www.chsrf.ca/final_research/ogc/pdf/davies_final_e.pdf.

Denis, J.L., Herbert, Y., Langley, A., Lozeau, D., & Tottier, L.H. (2002). Explaining diffusion patterns for complex health care innovations. *Health Care Management Review*, 27(3), 60–73.

Denis, J.L., Langley, A., & Rouleau, L. (2007). Strategizing in pluralistic contexts: Rethinking theoretical frames. *Human Relations*, 60(1), 179–215.

DiCenso, A., Guyatt, G., & Ciliska, D. (2005). *Evidence-Based Nursing: A Guide to Clinical Practice*. Philadelphia: Elsevier Mosby.

Duffy, A. (2007). A concept analysis of reflective practice: Determining its value to nurses. *British Journal of Nursing*, 16(22), 1400–1407.

Edwards, N. & Roelofs, S. (2006). Developing management systems with cross-cultural fit: Assessing international differences in operational systems. *International Journal of Health Planning and Management*, 21(1), 55–73.

Ferlie, E., Fitzgerald, L., Wood, M., & Hawkins, C. (2005). The non-spread of innovations: The mediating role of professionals. *Academy of Management Journal*, 48(1), 117–134.

Gifford, W. A., Davies, B., Edwards, N., & Graham, I.D. (2006). Leadership strategies to influence the use of clinical practice guidelines. *Nursing Leadership*, 19(4), 72–88.

Glasgow, R.E. & Emmons, K.M. (2007). How can we increase translation of research into practice? Types of evidence needed. *Annual Review of Public Health*, 28, 413–433.

Graham, I.D., Logan, J., Davies, B., & Nimrod, C. (2004). Changing the use of electronic fetal monitoring and labor support: A case study of barriers and facilitators. *Birth*, 31(4), 293–301.

Graham, I.D., Tetroe, J., & the KT Theories Research Group. (2007). Some theoretical underpinnings of knowledge translation. *Academic Emergency Medicine*, 14(11), 936–941.

Greenberg, A., Angus, H., Sullivan, T., & Brown, A.D. (2005). Development of a set of strategy-based system-level cancer care performance indicators in Ontario, Canada. *International Journal for Quality in Health Care*, 17(2), 107–114.

Greenhalgh, T., Robert, G., Bate, P., MacFarlane, F., & Kyriakidou, O. (2005). *Diffusion of Innovations in Health Service Organisations: A Systematic Literature Review*. Massachusetts: Blackwell Publishing, BMJ Books.

Hawe, P., Shiell, A., & Riley, T. (2004). Complex interventions: How "out of control" can a randomised controlled trial be? *British Medical Journal*, 328, 1561–1563.

Health Professions Regulatory Advisory Council. (2008). *Interprofessional collaboration. A summary of key reference documents & selected highlights from the literature*. Retrieved March 16, 2008, from http://www.hprac.org/en/projects/resources/hprac-collaboration.LitReviewENFINAL.feb1208.pdf.

Hodnett, E.D., Gates, S., Hofmeyr, G.J., & Sakala, C. (2007). Continuous support for women during childbirth. *Cochrane Database of Systematic Reviews*, 3, CD003766. DOI:10.1002/14651858.CD003766.pub2

Landry, R., Lamari, M, & Amara, N. (2003). The extent and determinants of the utilization of university research in government agencies. *Public Administration Review*, 63(2), 192–205.

Lind, C. & Smith, D. (2008). Analyzing the state of community health nursing advancing from deficit to strengths-based practice using appreciative inquiry. *Advances in Nursing Science*, 31(1), 28–41.

Maher, L., Gustafson, D., & Evans, A. (2007). Sustainability model and guide. NHS institute for innovation and improvement. Retrieved January 10, 2008, from www.institute.nhs.uk/sustainability.

Mann, K., Gordon, J., & MacLeod, A. (2007). Reflection and reflective practice in health professions education: A systematic review. *Advances in Health Sciences Education*, Published online: November, 23, 2007.

Mantzoukas, S. & Watkinson, S. (2008). Redescribing reflective practice and evidence-based practice discourses. *International Journal of Nursing Practice*, 14(2), 129–134.

Marchionni, C. & Richer, M. (2007). Using appreciative inquiry to promote evidence-based practice in nursing: The glass is more than half full. *Canadian Journal of Nursing Leadership*, 20(3), 86–97.

McWilliam, C. (2007). Continuing education at the cutting edge: Promoting transformative knowledge translation. *Journal of Continuing Education in the Health Professions*, 27(2), 72–79.

McWilliam, C., Kothari, A., Ward-Griffin, C., Forbes, D., Leipert, B., & South West Community Care Access Centre Home Care Collaboration (SW-CCAC). (2009). Evolving the theory and praxis of knowledge translation through social interaction: A social phenomenological study. *Implementation Science*, 4, 26.

Meagher, D., Edwards, N., Aston, M., & Young, L. (2009). Population health surveillance practice of public health nurses. *Public Health Nursing*, 26(6), 553–560.

National Leadership and Innovation Agency for Healthcare Sustainability Model. (2009). Excel Spreadsheet Updated April 3, 2009. Retrieved June 15, 2009, from http://www.wales.nhs.uk/sitesplus/ 829/page/36527.

NHS Institute for Innovation and Improvement. (2007). Improvement leaders' guide: Sustainability and its relationship with spread and adoption. Retrieved January 10, 2009, from www.institute.nhs.uk/sustainability.

Nutley, S.M., Walter, I., & Davies, H.T.O. (2007). *Using Evidence: How Research Can Inform Public Services*. Bristol: The Policy Press..

Oandasan, I., Baker, G.R., Barker, K. et al. (2006). Teamwork in healthcare: Promoting effective teamwork in healthcare in Canada. Retrieved April 22, 2009, from http://www.chsrf.ca/research_themes/ pdf/teamwork-synthesis-report_e.pdf.

Ontario Perinatal Partnership Program. (2006). Provincial Perinatal Report. Retrieved January 10, 2009, from http://www.pppeso.on.ca/site/ pppeso/NIDAY_Perinatal_Database_p484.html.

Paget, P. (2001). Reflective practice and clinical outcomes: Practitioners' views on how reflective practice has influenced their clinical practice. *Journal of Clinical Nursing*, 10(2), 204–214.

Perinatal Partnership Program of Eastern and South-eastern Ontario. (2008). Annual Perinatal Statistical Report 2007–2008. Retrieved January 10, 2009, from http://www.pppeso.on.ca/site/pppeso/NIDAY_ Perinatal_Database_p484.html.

Pluye, P., Potvin, L., & Denis, J.-L. (2004). Making public health programs last: Conceptualizing sustainability. *Evaluation and Program Planning*, 27, 121–133.

Potvin, L. & Golberg, C. (2006). Deux rôles joués par l'évaluation dans la transformation de la pratique en promotion de la santé. In: M. O'Neil, S. Dupere, A. Pederson, & I. Rootman (eds) *Promotion de la santé au Canada et au Québec, Perspectives Critiques*. Québec: Presses de l'Université Laval, pp. 457–473.

Reay, T., Golden-Biddle, K., & Germann, K. (2003). Challenges and leadership strategies for managers of nurse practitioners. *Journal of Nursing Management*, 11(6), 396–403.

Registered Nurses' Association of Ontario (RNAO) (2002). Toolkit: Implementation of clinical guidelines—Registered Nurses' Association of Ontario, Toronto, Canada. Retrieved September 4, 2008, from http://www.rnao.org/Storage/12/668_BPG_Toolkit.pdf.

Registered Nurses' Association of Ontario (RNAO) (2006). Collaborative practice among nursing teams—Registered Nurses' Association of Ontario, Toronto, Canada. Retrieved December 15, 2006, from http://www.rnao.org/Storage/23/1776_BPG_Collaborative_Practice.pdf.

Registered Nurses' Association of Ontario (RNAO) (2008). Nursing best practice guidelines. Retrieved October 20, 2008, from http://www.rnao.org/Page.asp?PageID=861&SiteNodeID=133.

Rogers, E.M. (2003). *Diffusion of Innovations*, 5th ed. New York: Free Press.

Rolfe, G. (2005). The deconstructing angel: Nursing, reflection and evidence-based practice. *Nursing Inquiry*, 12(2), 78–86.

Sandywell, B. (1996). *Reflexivity and the Crisis of Western Reason: Logological Investigations*, Vol. 1. London: Routledge.

Schön, D. (1983). *The Reflective Practitioner How Professionals Think in Action*. London: Temple Smith.

Shediac-Rizkallah, M.C. & Bone, L.R. (1998). Planning for the sustainability of community-based health programs: Conceptual frameworks and future directions for research, practice and policy. *Health Education Research*, 13(1), 87–108.

Sibbald, S., Singer, P., Upshur, R., & Martin, D. (2009). Priority setting: What constitutes success? A conceptual framework for successful priority setting. *BMC Health Services Research*, 9, 43.

Sicotte, C., Champagne, F., Contandriopoulos, A.-P. et al. (1998). A conceptual framework for the analysis of health care organizations' performance. *Health Services Management Research*, 11(1), 24–41.

Sitzia, J., Cotterell, P., & Richardson, A. (2006). Interprofessional collaboration with service users in the development of cancer services: The cancer partnership project. *Journal of Interprofessional Care*, 20(1), 60–74.

Thomas, L.H., McColl, E., Cullum, N., Rousseau, N., Soutter, J., & Steen, N. (1998). Effect of clinical guidelines in nursing, midwifery, and the therapies: A systematic review of evaluations. *Quality in Health Care*, 7(4), 183–191.

Thornhill, J., Dault, M., & Clements, D. (2008). CHSRF knowledge transfer: Ready, set… collaborate? The evidence says "go," so what's slowing adoption of inter-professional collaboration in primary healthcare? *Healthcare Quarterly*, 11(2), 14–16.

Watkins, C., Timm, A., Gooberman-Hill, R., Harvey, I., Haines, A., & Donovan, J. (2004). Factors affecting feasibility and acceptability of a practice-based educational intervention to support evidence-based prescribing: a qualitative study. *Family Practice*, 21(6), 661–669.

Wensing, M. & Grol, R. (2005). *Improving Patient Care: The Implementation of Change in Clinical Practice*. New York: Elsevier.

# Chapter 10

# A review of the use of outcome measures of evidence-based practice in guideline implementation studies in Nursing, Allied Health Professions, and Medicine

*Christina M. Godfrey, Margaret B. Harrison, and Ian D. Graham*

---

**Key learning points**

- Study outcomes reflect the effectiveness of implementation strategies.
- Diversity of outcomes and methods to measure them complicates comparison of implementation studies.
- Provider's instrumental use of knowledge (action taken with the knowledge) is most frequently measured.
- Further research is needed on the impact of providers' behavior indicating the effect at the patient level.

Research to determine the effectiveness of strategies to implement evidence-based practice (EBP) and enhance the quality of care is steadily increasing. However, to evaluate the effectiveness of these strategies we need to examine the outcomes that are measured as indicators of success or failure of these efforts. The variety of outcomes that are measured plus the diversity of methods used to measure these outcomes complicate comparison between implementation studies and may be hindering the adoption of strategies at the local level. We need to compare both intervention strategies and outcome measurements to make meaningful conclusions about which strategies or combinations of strategies can be relied upon to consistently and efficiently achieve successful outcomes.

This chapter focuses on the measurement of outcomes within the context of implementation research. Studies contributing to this context have investigated strategies for implementing clinical guidelines in practice. The current knowledge on guideline dissemination and implementation strategies indicates that there is no clear-cut formula, no specific strategy or even set of strategies that can be relied upon to successfully and consistently implement guidelines into practice (Grimshaw et al. 2004; Harrison et al. 2010). Examining the outcome measures used in practice guideline implementation studies offers insight into the diversity of outcome measurement in EBP and indicates the value and difficulty of comparing outcomes between implementation studies.

To explore outcome measurement we adopt the framework of knowledge use and its impact proposed by Graham and colleagues (see Chapter 2), and the categorization of methods of measurement proposed by Hakkennes and Green (2006). These approaches are examined using the outcome measures reported by two systematic reviews on implementing clinical practice guidelines in practice, using studies focused on nursing, allied health, and medicine (Grimshaw et al. 2004; Harrison et al. 2010). In this chapter we compare and discuss what outcomes were measured, how the outcomes were measured and illustrate differences with regard to these different professional groups (Table 10.1).

## Method and background on the reviews

Grimshaw and colleagues (Grimshaw et al. 2004) performed a systematic review on the dissemination strategies to implement guidelines

**Table 10.1** Classification of outcome measures according to Hakkennes and Green (2006) and Graham and colleagues (Chapter 2)

| Hakkennes and Green (2006) | Graham and colleagues (Chapter 2) |
| --- | --- |
| A. Patient level | |
| 1. Measurements of actual change in health status, i.e., pain, depression, mortality, and quality of life | Impact of knowledge use—Effect from applying the knowledge, i.e., changes in health status |
| 2. Surrogate measures of A1, i.e., patient compliance, length of stay, patient attitudes | Knowledge use—Instrumental, i.e., changes in patient behavior |
| B. Practitioner | |
| 1. Measurement of actual change in health practice, i.e., compliance with guidelines, changes in prescribing rates | Knowledge use—Instrumental, i.e., changes in practice, adherence to EBP recommendations |
| 2. Surrogate measures of B1, such as health practitioner knowledge and attitudes | Knowledge use—Conceptual, i.e., changes in knowledge, attitudes, intentions |
| C. Organizational or process level | |
| Measurement of change in the health system (i.e., wait lists), change in policy, costs, and usability and/or extent of the intervention | • Knowledge use—Surrogate measures of instrumental use, i.e., changes in policies, staffing, acquiring equipment |
| | • Impact of knowledge use—Effect from applying the knowledge, i.e., changes in expenditure, resource use, wait times, length of stay, visits to emergency department, hospitalizations and readmissions |

Outcomes measures (Hakkennes & Green 2006: p. 3).

in medicine. Their comprehensive search of the literature (1966–1998) located 235 studies and included only the most rigorous research designs (randomized controlled trials, controlled clinical trials, controlled before and after studies, and interrupted time series studies). Results from this review are taken from the included studies only, all of which report an "objective" measure of provider behavior. Survey-based measures at the level of provider (intention) are excluded from the review.

The outcomes measured by these studies were reanalyzed by Hakkennes and Green (2006: pp. 3,4) and allocated to nine categories of outcome measurement:

- Medical record audit,
- Computerized medical record audit,

- Health practitioner survey/questionnaire/interview,
- Patient survey/questionnaire/interview,
- Computerized database (pharmacy prescription registers; medical billing information),
- Log books/department record/register (emergency department visit records; log books of X-ray requests),
- Encounter chart/request slips/diary (data collection forms designed by the study and completed by practitioners; diaries for study data collection),
- Other (laboratory tests, audio/video taping of consultations), and
- Unclear (method of measurement not clear).

Hakkennes and Green (2006) also categorized the studies according to those that measured patient outcomes ($n = 155$); provider outcomes ($n = 242$), and system outcomes ($n = 87$).

In a similar fashion, the systematic review performed by Harrison and colleagues (2009) focused on the guideline dissemination and implementation strategies in nursing and allied health professions. Their expansive search of the literature (1995–2007) located 53 studies (36 nursing, 17 allied health). They also included only the most rigorous research designs (randomized controlled trials and controlled before and after studies). Included studies in this review report both "objective" measures of provider behavior as well as intention to act. The outcomes measured by these studies were analyzed according to the nine categories proposed by Hakkennes and Green (2006), and tallied into patient outcomes (nursing: $n = 15$; allied health: $n = 8$); provider outcomes (nursing $n = 30$; allied health: $n = 16$); and system outcomes (nursing: $n = 11$; allied health: $n = 9$).

The outcomes of both reviews were then classified according to the categories of knowledge use or the impact of knowledge use. Knowledge use is divided into *conceptual use* which refers to the knowledge, attitudes, or intensions; and *instrumental use* which refers to behavior based on that knowledge. Impact of knowledge use is divided into *direct effects* resulting from applying the guidelines, such as changes in health status (patient) or changes in quality or continuity of care (provider); and *surrogate effects* of applying the guidelines, such as changes in return to work status (patient) or changes in job satisfaction (provider). Information from guideline implementation studies in medicine was obtained from the published data reported in the study by Hakkennes and Green (2006); however, in some cases, data from this study were not directly comparable or available. In these instances comparison is made between nursing and allied health and the lack of data for medicine is noted.

## Knowledge use and impact of knowledge use

In keeping with Graham and colleagues' framework (see Chapter 2), we distinguish between the use of knowledge and the impact of knowledge use. For example, measuring a provider's knowledge about pain management would be a measure of conceptual knowledge use (not action). Assessing the extent to which providers' follow pain guideline recommendations about pain assessment and management (i.e., adhere to the guideline) would be a measure of *instrumental* knowledge use (action, and behavior). Measuring a change in the patient's pain (i.e., assessing the effect of the pain management on that patient's pain) would be a measure of the *impact* of using the guideline. If the patient is pain free and consequently is able to return to work or to remain at work for several hours, this would be a measure of the surrogate effect of applying the guideline.

For nursing and allied health professions, many more of the guideline implementation studies reported knowledge use as an outcome measure compared to the impact of knowledge use (Table 10.2). Ninety-four percent of nursing studies and 100% of allied health

**Table 10.2** Proportion of guideline implementation studies with knowledge or impact outcome measures by profession

| | Nursing (*n* = 36) | Allied health (*n* = 17) | Medicine (*n* = 228) |
|---|---|---|---|
| Knowledge use | 34 (94%) | 17 (100%) | Not available |
| • Conceptual | 17 (47%) | 9 (53%) | 40 (18%) |
| • Instrumental | 32 (89%) | 17 (100%) | 227 (99%) |
| • Enabling knowledge use | 2 (5%) | 1 (6%) | Not available |
| Impact | 24 (67%) | 11 (65%) | 121 (53%) |
| • Effect from applying knowledge use | 23 (64%) | 11 (65%) | 95 (42%) |
| • Surrogate effect from applying knowledge use | 3 (8%) | 4 (24%) | 26 (11%) |

studies measured change in terms of knowledge use compared to 67% and 65% for impact of knowledge use respectively. For the studies in medicine, no data were available on the overall proportion of studies that included a measure of knowledge use; however, 53% of the studies measured impact of knowledge use.

Knowledge use comprises conceptual use, instrumental use, and enabling knowledge use. We see that it is the instrumental use of knowledge—the action taken with the knowledge that was measured most frequently; nursing 89%, allied health 100%, and medicine 99%. By comparison, measurement of the impact of that behavior is substantially lower for all three professional groups; nursing 64%, allied health 65%, and medicine 42%. Advancement of implementation research requires an increase in the measurement of impact of knowledge use to confirm that changes occurring at the provider behavior level have a significant change on the health status of patients; potential impact on providers; and appropriate adjustments at the system level.

## Knowledge use by provider and methods of measurement

The measure of providers' instrumental use of knowledge (providers' use of knowledge and adherence to guidelines) was the most common measurement in all three professional groups: nursing 30/36 (83%); allied health 16/17 (94%); medicine 213/228 (93%). However, applying Hakkennes and Greens' (2006) nine categories of measurement, the method of measuring providers' instrumental use of knowledge differed for each professional group (Table 10.3).

The most common method for both nursing and medicine was medical record audits (50% and 45% respectively). For allied health, provider surveys/questionnaire/interviews were the most common with 50% of the outcomes measured in this way. It is interesting to note that provider surveys/questionnaire/interviews were the least frequent method of measuring this outcome for medicine (5%), but are the second most frequent method for nursing (40%). As this measure is an indication of providers' adherence to guidelines, we see that patient surveys/questionnaire/interviews are also frequently used to assess these outcomes. For both nursing and allied health this measure is the third most frequent measure at 23% and 19% respectively. However, for medicine, querying the patient

**Table 10.3** Method used to assess providers instrumental use of knowledge by profession

|  | Nursing (*n*=36) | Allied health (*n*=17) | Medicine (*n*=228) |
| --- | --- | --- | --- |
| Medical record audit | 50% | 31% | 45% |
| Computerized medical record audit | 7% |  | 12% |
| Provider survey/questionnaire/interview | 40% | 50% | 5% |
| Patient survey/questionnaire/ interview | 23% | 19% | 10% |
| Computerized database | 7% | 6% | 25% |
| Log book/department record/register |  | 6% | 9% |
| Encounter chart/request slip/diary | 10% | 38% | 13% |
| Other | 17% | 6% | 7% |
| Unclear |  |  | 7% |

All numbers are percentages of the total number of studies for the categories: patient, provider, and system.

about doctors' behavior is only fifth in line as a potential method of measurement.

To assess the level of providers' knowledge the most common method used by all professional groups was provider surveys/ questionnaire/interviews, with nursing 37%, allied health 44%, and medicine 100%.

## Knowledge use by patient and methods of measurement

Comparing the measurement of the patients' conceptual use of knowledge (changes in the patients' knowledge, attitudes, or intentions), we see that the use of patient surveys/questionnaire/interviews is the most common method of measurement for both nursing and allied health (20% and 13% respectively). There were no data available for medicine. The patients' instrumental use of knowledge (changes in patients' behavior and/or adherence to evidence-based recommendations), also relied heavily on this method for both nursing and allied health (27% and 25% respectively) but for medicine, the medical record audit was the most commonly used measure of this outcome (29%).

# Impact of knowledge use by provider and methods of measurement

Measuring provider impact of knowledge use and effect from applying the knowledge (time spent doing EBP, the increase in quality of care and the continuity of care provided), we see that for nursing, provider surveys/questionnaire/interviews were the most common method with 20% of nursing studies measuring this outcome in this manner. For allied health however, 13% of studies measured this effect either by medical record audit, provider surveys/questionnaire/ interviews, patient surveys/questionnaire/interviews, or by encounter chart/request slip/diary methods. There were no data available for medicine.

# Impact of knowledge use by patient and methods of measurement

Each professional group measured patient impact of knowledge use and effect from applying the knowledge in a variety of ways (Table 10.4). This measure assesses patients' health status, function,

**Table 10.4** Method used to assess patient impact of knowledge use and effect of applying knowledge by profession

|  | Nursing (*n* = 36) | Allied health (*n* = 17) | Medicine (*n* = 228) |
|---|---|---|---|
| Medical record audit | 7% | 13% | 32% |
| Computerized medical record audit |  |  | 14% |
| Provider survey/questionnaire/Interview |  |  | 12% |
| Patient survey/questionnaire/Interview | 80% | 63% | 37% |
| Computerized database | 7% |  | 18% |
| Log book/department record/register | 7% |  | 2% |
| Encounter chart/request slip/diary | 7% | 13% | 8% |
| Other | 13% | 13% | 14% |
| Unclear | 7% |  | 9% |

All numbers are percentages of the total number of studies for the categories: patient, provider, and system.

morbidity, mortality, and quality of life. The most common methods of measurement were patient surveys/questionnaire/interviews (nursing 80%, allied health 63%, and medicine 37%), with medicine using the full range of other methods for this assessment.

## Impact of knowledge use by system and methods of measurement

Nursing, allied health, and medicine studies used a range of methods to measure system impact and effect of applying the knowledge on the system. These outcomes measure resource use, wait time, length of stay, visits to emergency departments, hospitalizations, and readmissions (Table 10.5).

For nursing, the most popular methods are medical record audits, computerized databases, and log book/departmental record/register (27%). For allied health, medical record audit was the most common (44%) and for medicine, provider surveys/questionnaire/interviews were the most frequently used method (53%). Given the range of system outcomes, this variety of measurement methods is not surprising.

**Table 10.5** Method used to assess impact of knowledge use on the system by profession

|  | Nursing (*n* = 36) | Allied health (*n* = 17) | Medicine (*n* = 228) |
|---|---|---|---|
| Medical record audit | 27% | 44% | 5% |
| Computerized medical record audit |  |  | 1% |
| Provider survey/questionnaire/interview | 18% |  | 53% |
| Patient survey/questionnaire/interview | 9% | 11% | 5% |
| Computerized database | 27% | 11% | 8% |
| Log book/department record/register | 27% |  | 6% |
| Encounter chart/request slip/diary |  | 22% | 13% |
| Other |  | 33% | 8% |
| Unclear |  |  | 6% |

All numbers are percentages of the total number of studies for the categories: patient, provider and system.

**Table 10.6** Most frequent methods of measurement by profession

| Nursing (*n*=36) | Allied health (*n*=17) | Medicine (*n*=228) |
|---|---|---|
| Patient survey/questionnaire/ interview (50%) | Provider survey/questionnaire/ interview (59%) | Medical record audit (51%) |
| Provider survey/questionnaire/ interview (47%) | Encounter chart/request slip/diary (53%) | Computerized database (31%) |
| Medical record audit (44%) | Patient survey/questionnaire/ interview (41%) | Provider survey/questionnaire/ interview (30%) |

## Methods of measurement

The most frequent methods of measurement differ by professional group (Table 10.6). Notably, there is a variety in the top three methods, patient or provider survey/questionnaire/interview and medical record audit. For a complete list of methods used to collect data for the different outcome measure categories see Appendix: Table A1 – nursing, Table A2 – allied health, Table A3 – medicine.

## Validity and reliability of measurements

When measuring outcomes, 19 (53%) of nursing studies, 5 (29%) of allied health studies, and 32 (14%) of medicine studies used or referenced at least one previously developed scale and/or questionnaire. Twenty-nine medicine studies assessed the reliability of the medical record audit—an assessment not performed in any of the nursing or allied health studies. However, two nursing studies based the extraction of data from medical records according to established guidelines of care.

When no preexisting scales were available, some studies indicated the assessment of validity and reliability of their own researcher developed scales. A total of 10 nursing studies (28%), 4 allied health studies (24%), and 46 medicine studies (20%) reported these activities, usually using pilots with experts and researchers.

## Discussion

In this chapter we focused on the range of outcomes in guideline implementation studies and what methods were used to capture them. The synopsis is drawn from two recent reviews in nursing, allied health, and medicine (Grimshaw et al. 2004; Harrison et al. 2010). Implementation research is occurring with many provider groups and the studies range across the continuum of health care. Not surprisingly the strategies used to initiate change in these settings also vary widely. We have seen how studies in nursing, allied health, and medicine approach the measurement of outcomes differently both in terms of what concepts are measured as well as how these concepts are measured.

Measurement of providers' instrumental use of knowledge (providers' use of knowledge and adherence to guidelines) was the most common measurement in all three professional groups, with both medicine and nursing using an audit of medical records to assess this outcome (50% and 45% respectively) and allied health groups using provider surveys/questionnaire/interviews (50%).

The current knowledge in implementation research reflects the need to understand which strategies are successful at increasing the use of guidelines in practice and which settings are the most appropriate for or would benefit the most by each strategy or set of strategies. The array of outcomes being measured compounded by varying methods with which to measure them, make comparison across studies virtually impossible. Unfortunately this provides little direction or clarity about what best measurement practice might be from research and/or implementation perspective. The difficulty of adapting strategies to the local level is made all the more complex when faced with the multiplicity of outcomes and measurement methods. Although standardizing the use of common outcome measures would facilitate comparison across studies, the variety of practice settings and the need to adapt strategies to each setting precludes this restriction for implementation research (Hakkennes & Green 2006). However, identification of some common approaches to outcomes measurement would be a step in the right direction.

For example, the advancement of implementation research will benefit by consistent measurement of provider instrumental knowledge use and the reporting of the reliability and validity of data collection methods (Hakkennes & Green 2006). The most important advance would be increasing the measurement of impact of EBP, that is, knowledge use and the effect of applying knowledge on patient, provider, and the system, although this may increase both complexity and resources needed for research process. This would provide confirmation that the changes made in provider or patient behavior have an impact and ultimately improve patient health status.

## Conclusion

To advance the science of implementation research we are striving for consensus and consistency in the measurement of study outcomes. However, two large reviews focused on medicine, nursing, and allied health professions and covering a total of 286 implementation studies indicate that not only are we far from agreement on common methods of measurement, there are disparate views as to what elements need to be measured. It is clear that currently, the instrumental use of knowledge (providers' action taken with the knowledge) is the most frequent measure. By comparison, measurement of the impact of the providers' behavior, and the indicator as to whether we are actually making a difference at the patient level, is substantially lower for all three professional groups. Uniformity of measure and consensus as to what are the indicators of success vis-a-vis the implementation of new knowledge would be most valuable at this time.

## References

Grimshaw, J.M., Thomas, R.E., MacLennan, G. et al. (2004). Effectiveness and efficiency of guideline dissemination and implementation strategies. *Health Technology Assessment*, 8(6), 1–84.

Hakkennes, S. & Green, S. (2006). Measures for assessing practice change in medical practitioners. *Implementation Science*, 1, 29–37.

Harrison, M.B., Graham, I.D., Godfrey, C.M. et al. (2010). Guideline dissemination and implementation strategies in Nursing and Allied Health Professions. *The Cochrane Collaboration* (under review).

# Appendix

**Table A1** Method used to collect for the different outcome measure categories for nursing (n = 36)

| | Patient n=15 n(%) | | | | | Provider n=30 n(%) | | | | | System n=11 n(%) | | |
|---|---|---|---|---|---|---|---|---|---|---|---|---|---|
| | Concept/ knowledge | Inst. use knowledge | Enable use knowledge | Effect | Surrogate effect | Concept/ knowledge | Inst. use knowledge | Enable use knowledge | Effect | Surrogate effect | Concept/ knowledge | Inst. use knowledge | Enable use knowledge |
| Medical record audit | | | | 1(7) | | 1(3) | 15(50) | | 5(17) | | | 3(27) | |
| Computerized medical record audit | | | | | | | 2(7) | | | | | | |
| Provider survey/ questionnaire/ interview | | | | | | 11(37) | 12(40) | | 6(20) | 1(3) | 1(9) | 2(18) | |
| Patient survey/ questionnaire/ interview | 3(20) | 4(27) | | 12(80) | 2(13) | 1(3) | 7(23) | | 5(17) | | | 1(9) | |
| Computerized database | | | | 1(7) | | | 2(7) | | | | | 3(27) | |
| Log book/ department record/register | | | | 1(7) | | | | | | | | 3(27) | |
| Encounter chart/request slip/diary | | | | 1(7) | | | 3(10) | 1(3) | 2(7) | | | | |
| Other | | | | 2(13) | | 1(3) | 5(17) | | | | | | |
| Unclear | | | | 1(7) | | | | | | | | | |

All numbers are percentages of the total number of studies for the categories: patient, provider, and system.

**Table A2** Method used to collect for the different outcome measure categories for allied health professionals (n = 17)

| | Patient (n=8) n(%) | | | | | Provider (n=16) n(%) | | | | | System (n=9) n(%) | | |
|---|---|---|---|---|---|---|---|---|---|---|---|---|---|
| | Concept/ knowledge | Inst. use knowledge | Enable use knowledge | Effect | Surrogate effect | Concept/ knowledge | Inst. use knowledge | Enable use knowledge | Effect | Surrogate effect | Concept/ knowledge | Inst. use knowledge | Enable use knowledge |
| Medical record audit | | | | 1(13) | | | 5(31) | | 2(13) | | | 4(44) | |
| Computerized medical record audit | | | | | | | | | | | | | |
| Provider survey/ questionnaire/ interview | | | | | | 7(44) | 8(50) | | 2(13) | | | | |
| Patient survey/ questionnaire/ interview | 1(13) | 2(25) | 1(13) | 5(63) | 8(100) | | 3(19) | | 2(13) | | | 1(11) | |
| Computerized database | | | | | | | 1(6) | | | | | 1(11) | |
| Log book/ department record/register | | | | | | | 1(6) | | | | | | |
| Encounter chart/request slip/diary | | 1(13) | | 1(13) | | 1(6) | 6(38) | | 2(13) | | | 2(22) | |
| Other | | | | 1(13) | | | 1(6) | | 1(6) | | | | |
| Unclear | | | | | | | | | | | | 3(33) | |

All numbers are percentages of the total number of studies for the categories: patient, provider, and system.

**Table A3** Method used to collect for the different outcome measure categories for medicine ($n = 228$)

| | Patient ($n=155$) (%) | | | | | Provider ($n=243$) (%) | | | | | System ($n=87$) (%) | | |
|---|---|---|---|---|---|---|---|---|---|---|---|---|---|
| | Concept/ knowledge | Inst. use knowledge | Enable use knowledge | Effect | Surrogate effect | Concept/ knowledge | Inst. use knowledge | Enable use knowledge | Effect | Surrogate effect | Concept/ knowledge | Inst. use knowledge | Enable use knowledge |
| Medical record audit | | (29) | | (32) | | | (45) | | | | | (5) | |
| Computerized medical record audit | | (9) | | (14) | | | (12) | | | | | (1) | |
| Provider survey/ questionnaire/ interview | | (2) | | (12) | | (100) | (5) | | | | | (53) | |
| Patient survey/ questionnaire/ interview | | (4) | | (37) | | | (10) | | | | | (5) | |
| Computerized database | | (26) | | (18) | | | (25) | | | | | (18) | |
| Log book/ department record/register | | (7) | | (2) | | | (9) | | | | | (6) | |
| Encounter chart/request slip/diary | | (3) | | (8) | | | (13) | | | | | (13) | |
| Other | | (7) | | (14) | | | (7) | | | | | (8) | |
| Unclear | | (14) | | (9) | | | (7) | | | | | (6) | |

All numbers are percentages of the total number of studies for the categories: patient, provider, and system.
*Source:* From Hakkennes and Green (2006); Table 3: p. 7. Numbers not available.

# Index